SLEEP APNEA IN CHILDREN: A HANDBOOK FOR FAMILIES

Edited by

DAVID INGRAM, MD

To Molly

Who reminds me that I'm nobody if I'm not trying to help somebody

CONTENTS

DAVID INGRAM, MD

ACKNOWLEDGMENTS

I want to thank my patients and their families, whose courage makes our work possible; my colleagues who contributed to this work and made this book happen; my many mentors and teachers in sleep medicine; our medical writing and legal teams at CMH; and most of all my wife and daughter, who make it all worthwhile.

SLEEP BASICS
Njideka L. Osuala, DNP, APRN

What is sleep?

Sleep is a fascinating process that we all should experience every day. We spend about a third of our lives asleep. Even so, we still have much to learn about exactly how sleep works and why it happens. Certainly, we recognize that when someone is asleep they have decreased interaction, less response to the surrounding environment, and reduced body movement. While we may think that the purpose of sleep is to "rest" the mind, the brain is actually extremely active during sleep. One thing is clear: our body and mind need sleep. Just as we feel more thirsty the longer we go without a drink of water, the longer we stay awake during the day, the more sleepy we start to feel.

There are two basic types of sleep: non-rapid eye movement (NREM) sleep and rapid eye movement (REM) sleep. Further, NREM sleep is divided into three stages.

Stage 1 sleep (N1) occurs as your child gets drowsy and is falling asleep. Since this is your child's lightest sleep stage, it is easy for him to wake up. His heartbeat, breathing, and eye movements slow down. His eyes start to move slowly back and forth with the eyelids closed. Muscles relax, and he may have occasional brief movements or jerks in the muscles in his arms and legs. When our eyelids get heavy and our head starts to slump while reading this book, we are likely falling into stage 1 sleep. Usually, stage 1 accounts for about 5%-10% of overall sleep.

During stage 2 sleep (N2), your child's sleep moves from a light to a slightly deeper state. Her heartbeat and breathing rate continue to decrease. Her muscles also relax further. Brain activity starts to show new large waves called "K-complexes" and smaller fast bursts called "sleep spindles." About 40%-55% of the night is spent in stage 2 sleep.

Stage 3 sleep (N3) is called "deep sleep," because it is the most difficult stage to wake up from. Your child's breathing and heartbeat are at their slowest rate during this stage. Her muscles are relaxed.

Brain activity shows large slow waves, called "delta waves," at this stage of sleep. Growth hormone is secreted from the brain during this stage. A sleeping child who doesn't wake easily is likely in stage 3 sleep. About 20%-30% of the night is spent in stage 3 sleep.

REM sleep (R) is when most dreaming occurs. During REM sleep, your child's eyes move rapidly from side to side under closed eyelids, similar to his eye movements when he is awake. In addition, his brain waves are similar to those when he is awake. Breathing and heart rate become more irregular. During REM sleep almost all of your child's muscles are actively paralyzed (except those of the eyes, ears, and breathing). This paralysis is for good reason. If muscles were not actively paralyzed, the dreamer would enact his dreams, as with the disorder known as REM behavior disorder. Sleep apnea tends to be worse during REM sleep because the muscles of the upper airway are relaxed and more prone to collapse, resulting in airway obstruction. About 15%-25% of the night is spent in REM sleep.

The figure below illustrates N1 sleep. The brain waves slow as the child becomes drowsy and shifts from wakefulness to stage 1 sleep. Note the change in EEG frequency and the development of slow rolling eye movements.

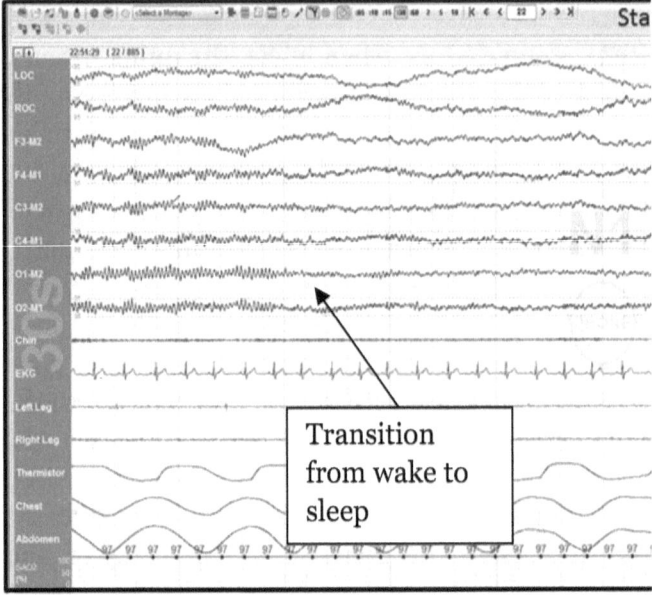

Transition from wake to sleep

The figure below shows an example of N2 sleep. Note the sleep spindles on EEG during this stage of sleep.

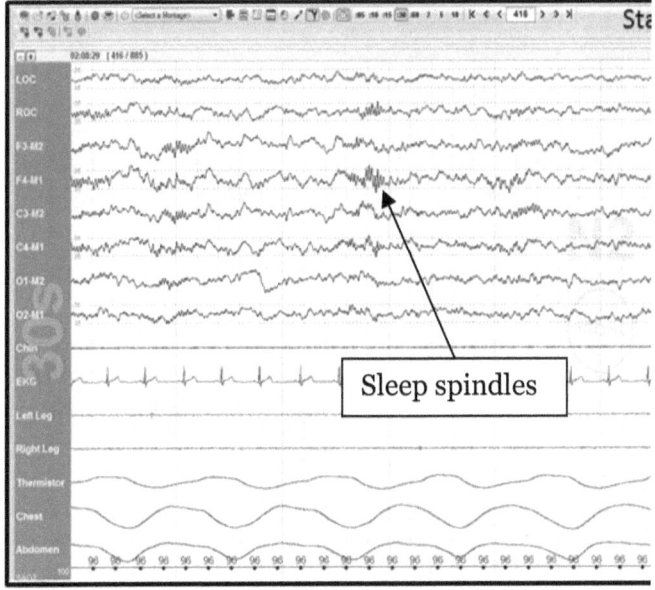

The figure below illustrates N3 sleep. There are large "delta waves" seen on EEG.

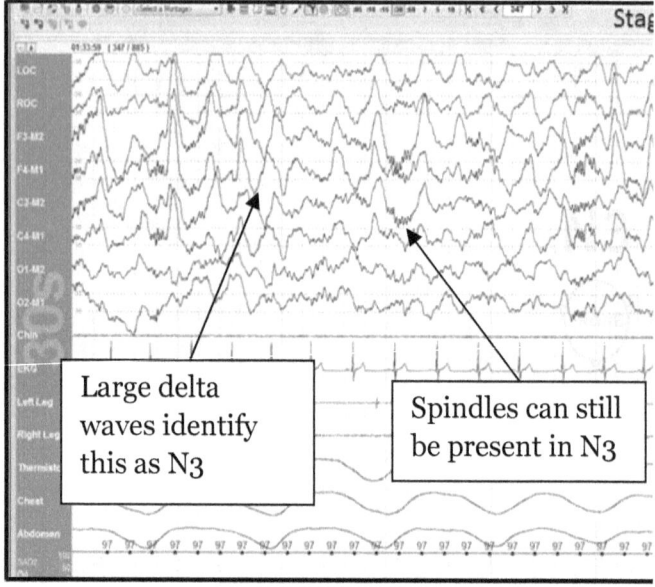

Large delta waves identify this as N3

Spindles can still be present in N3

The figure below illustrates REM sleep. There are frequent rapid eye movements, low chin muscle tone, and active EEG pattern.

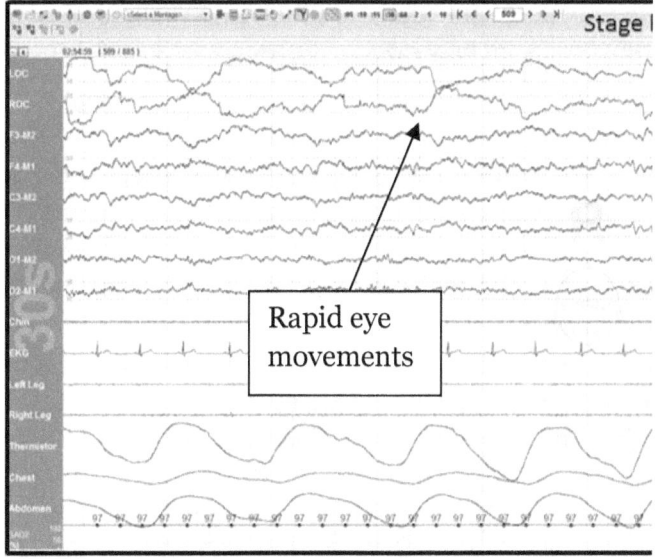

Rapid eye movements

What are sleep cycles?

During the course of the night, your child cycles between the different stages of sleep described above. Typically, she starts the night falling asleep into stage 1, then progresses to stage 2, then stage 3, and then REM. However, the cycles need not strictly follow that sequence and pattern. Over the course of the night, the duration of stage 3 sleep tends to decrease and REM sleep tends to increase. Each of these cycles lasts about 90-110 minutes, such that there are 4-6 cycles on a typical night. Sleep cycles vary dramatically depending on the age and development of a child. For instance, infants tend to enter into REM sleep almost immediately after falling asleep, having shorter sleep cycles that occur during the day and the night, and proportionally have a much greater amount of REM sleep. As children develop and age, they enter NREM instead of REM first, the sleep cycles lengthen and occur only at night, and the overall amount of REM sleep decreases.

The figure below shows a typical sequence of sleep cycles that a child progresses through during the night. Note that the child goes from wake to light sleep (N1 and N2), and then has a long period of deep sleep (N3) in the beginning third of the night. As the night progresses, REM sleep periods (black bars) increase slightly in duration. Night terrors and sleepwalking tend to occur out of N3 sleep and are more common in the beginning third of the night, whereas nightmares occur during REM sleep.

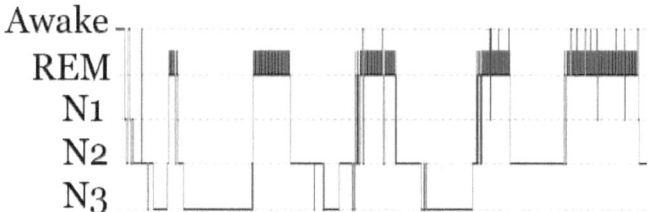

Why does my child sleep?

Healthy sleep is extremely important for the overall health of your child. Critical processes occur during sleep that help your child grow and develop normally. Growth hormone, released predominantly during stage 3 sleep[1], helps your child grow bigger and stronger, and assists with cell repair. Getting enough sleep helps keep the immune system functioning properly to protect your child from infections. For example, one study showed that sleep deprivation decreases the immune response to the flu vaccine[2]. Another study found that not getting enough sleep almost tripled the risk of catching the common cold when exposed to the virus[3]. Getting enough sleep also allows your child's brain to grow and develop, improves learning and memory, and helps her to reach her full potential in school. While we don't fully understand how sleep helps the brain at night, some research has found that neurotoxins and waste products that accumulate during the day are actually cleared from the fluid surrounding the brain during nighttime sleep[4]. Not getting enough sleep can cause your child to have behavior and mood problems during the day.

How much sleep does my child need?

Children grow and develop rapidly, and consequently need a greater amount of sleep than adults do. In addition, the need for sleep varies dramatically depending on a child's age. Finally, it is important to know that every child is different, and the right amount of sleep will vary, even for children of the same age. Most important is how your child is functioning during the day on a particular amount of sleep. You can think of this like shoe size: we all have slightly different sized feet, and we know we have the right shoe size when it feels right. General guidelines for sleep duration have been published by the National Sleep Foundation as well as the American Academy of Sleep Medicine.

Sleep duration recommendations from the American Academy of Sleep Medicine are as follows[5]:

- Infants 4-12 months of age: 12-16 hours (including naps)
- Children 1-2 years of age: 11-14 hours (including naps)
- Children 3-5 years of age: 10-13 hours (including naps)
- Children 6-12 years of age: 9-12 hours
- Teenagers 13-18 years of age: 8-10 hours

What are other common sleep disorders besides sleep apnea?

Insomnia is a sleep disorder in which children have trouble falling asleep or staying asleep at night. Insomnia can also make a child wake up too early in the morning. Symptoms of insomnia include irritability, decreased attention span, depression, and hyperactivity. It is estimated that about 29% of children ages 5-12 years and 9%-24% of adolescents have insomnia, based on parental report[6].

Restless legs syndrome (RLS), also known as Willis-Ekbom disease, is best described as a strong urge to move the legs, usually accompanied by an uncomfortable feeling felt in the lower legs. It can be hard for younger children to describe the feeling of RLS. Some children have described RLS symptoms as "bugs crawling on my legs" or "funny feelings" in the legs. Some children may even complain of their legs "hurting" at bedtime. Parents often report having to rub their child's legs to make them feel better. About 1.5 million children and adolescents have RLS in the United States[6].

Periodic limb movement disorder (PLMD) is a neurological disorder that occurs during sleep. It involves a series of repetitive movements, usually in the legs. They occur at about 20-40 second intervals. The movements may happen quickly and look like muscle twitches or jerking movements. Movement from PLMD can cause frequent awakenings during the night, which in turn causes children to be tired during the day. RLS is related to PLMD, and many children and adolescents with RLS have frequent periodic leg movements. Infants and young children may be diagnosed first with PLMD and then with RLS when they are older and better able to communicate the leg symptoms. Many times, parents will report that their children move their legs a lot during sleep, or that their children have restless or unrefreshing sleep. A sleep study is required to diagnose PLMD.

Delayed sleep-wake phase disorder (DSWPD) is a sleep problem that can occur at any age but is most common in teenagers and young adults. Those with DSWPD have a preference for staying up late and sleeping into the late morning, especially on weekends, holidays, and vacations. The usual sleep-wake pattern in those with DSWPD is a preferred bedtime after midnight (typically 2-6 a.m.) and wake time after 10 a.m. Children and teens who are natural "night owls" are more likely to develop DSWPD, which causes problems with everyday activities such as school. An estimated 7%-16% of adolescents have DSWPD[6]. A teen with DSWPD wants to go to bed earlier, but cannot, unlike a teen who chooses to stay up later. Signs of DSWPD are inability to wake up at the desired time and daytime sleepiness. Children and teens with DSWPD usually have no other sleep complaints and sleep well.

Nightmares are scary dreams that usually result in waking up from sleep. Nightmares happen more often during a difficult time, such as a child's parent being away overnight, or a child starting at a new school. Some children have nightmares about traumatic events they have gone through, such as getting shots, or about a scary movie they watched.

Children or teens who have nightmares will be able to remember the nightmare and describe it. Nightmares are common, with approximately 75% of children having at least one nightmare in their life[6].

Sleep terrors, also called "night terrors," are most common in young children. A child having a sleep terror will often cry or scream and appear confused, scared, or upset. A sleep terror can be frightening for caregivers to watch, but it is important to know that the child is unaware of his behavior or what is happening, because he is deeply asleep. Also, sleep terrors are not nightmares. Sleep terrors can last for 5-10 minutes. About 1%-6.5% of children have sleep terrors, which typically begin between the ages of 4 and 12 years[6].

Sleepwalking is common in children, and occurs during the first few hours of the night. Children who are sleepwalking may look awake, but they are actually sleeping. They may look confused and may even mumble or give strange answers if asked a question. A sleepwalking child may leave the home or do strange things, such as urinate in the closet. It is important that the area be kept safe around where a sleepwalking child sleeps. No sharp objects should be near and the ground should be clear. Sleepwalking is not harmful, and children usually grow out of it by the time they are teenagers. Between 15% and 40% of children sleepwalk at least once[6].

References

1. Van Cauter E, Plat L. Physiology of growth hormone secretion during sleep. J Pediatr. 1996 May;128(5 Pt 2):S32-7.
2. Spiegel K, Sheridan JF, Van Cauter E. Effect of sleep deprivation on response to immunization. JAMA. 2002 Sep 25;288(12):1471-2.
3. Cohen S, Doyle WJ, Alper CM, et al. Sleep habits and susceptibility to the common cold. Arch Intern Med. 2009 Jan 12;169(1):62-7.
4. Xie L, Kang H, Xu Q, et al. Sleep drives metabolite clearance from the adult brain. Science. 2013;342(6156):373.
5. Paruthi S, Brooks LJ, D'Ambrosio C, et al. Recommended Amount of Sleep for Pediatric Populations: A Consensus Statement of the American Academy of Sleep Medicine. J Clin Sleep Med. 2016 Jun 15;12(6):785-6.
6. Mindell, J. A., Owens, J. A. (2015). A clinical guide to pediatric sleep diagnosis and management of sleep problems 3rd edition. Philadelphia, PA: Lippincott Williams & Wilkins.

2

UNDERSTANDING SLEEP APNEA
Bahauddin A. Al-Shawwa, MD

What is sleep apnea?

Sleep apnea is an involuntary pause of air movement through the nose or the mouth for an extended period of time that occurs only during sleep. A complete stoppage of air movement is called an "apnea." However, patients frequently have partial stoppage of air movement, or a shallow breath, which is called a "hypopnea." Both apneas and hypopneas contribute to sleep apnea and therefore both are potentially harmful.

There are three types of apnea: obstructive, central, and mixed. An obstructive apnea occurs when the patient tries to breathe by moving his chest and abdomen, but there is no airflow through the nose or the mouth due to blockage in the upper airway.

The figure below illustrates an obstructive apnea recorded during a sleep study. There is an absence of airflow from the nose and mouth, even though the child is still trying to breathe (the chest and abdomen are moving). This apnea also results in an arousal (awakening) from sleep. Notice that snoring is seen leading up to the apnea, stops when airflow stops, and resumes with an awakening.

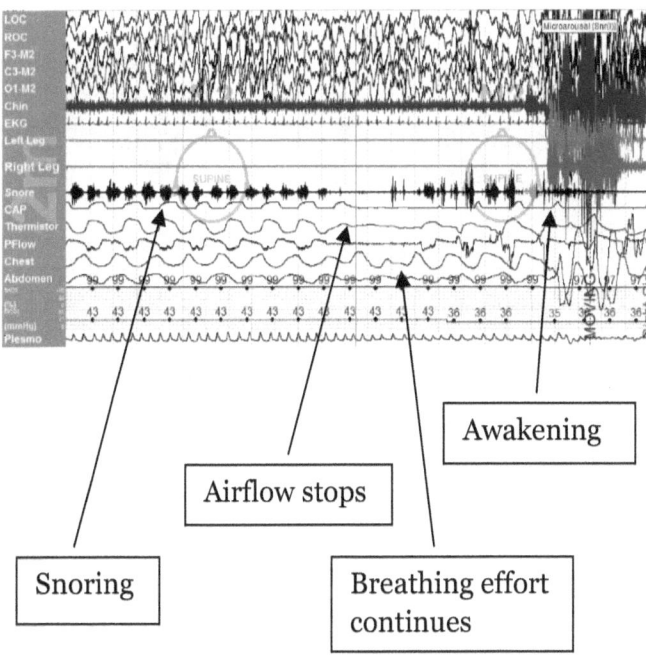

In contrast, a central apnea occurs when the patient lacks the signal from the brain to breathe; therefore there is no effort to move the chest or the abdomen, which leads to a lack of airflow through the nose or the mouth. Finally, a mixed apnea occurs when the apnea starts as a central apnea but then switches midway through to become obstructive. In general, mixed apneas are regarded as primarily due to airway obstruction, and usually lumped together with obstructive apneas.

The figure below illustrates a central apnea. Notice the lack of snoring and respiratory effort.

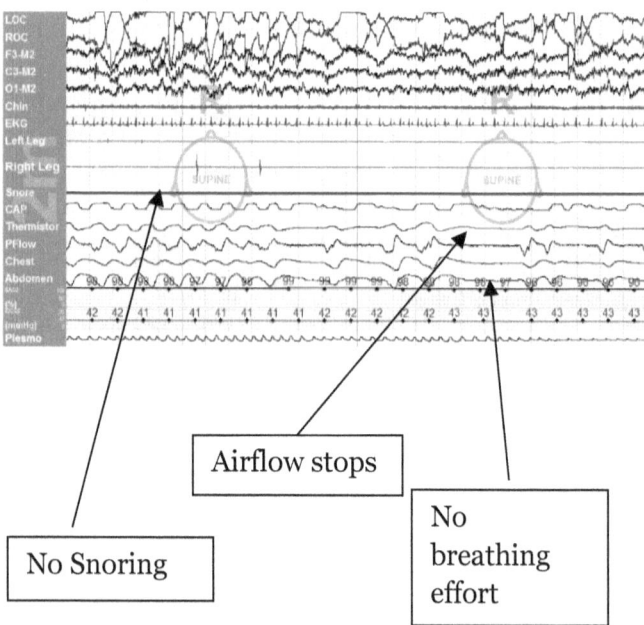

Airflow stops

No breathing effort

No Snoring

While everyone has occasional apneas or hypopneas during sleep, if they are frequent enough they can disrupt sleep and contribute to a host of potential health problems, as described below. Therefore, when frequent apneas and hypopneas are noted on a sleep study, this is considered a disease and the medical diagnosis of sleep apnea can be made. When the majority of apneas and hypopneas are obstructive, the diagnosis is obstructive sleep apnea (OSA). When the majority of apneas and hypopneas are central, the diagnosis is central sleep apnea (CSA).

What causes sleep apnea?

Causes of sleep apnea differ depending on what type of sleep apnea the patient has. Obstructive sleep apnea occurs due to complete or partial blockage of the upper airway (the nose, tongue, and throat). In children, a frequent cause of upper airway obstruction is enlarged tonsils or adenoids. However, other possible reasons for airway obstruction are obesity, birth defects, small jaw, large tongue, or neuro-muscular weakness. During sleep, the throat muscles relax and the tongue can fall backward, which can lead to complete or partial blockage of the upper airway that may already be small due to the reasons mentioned above. This in turn decreases or blocks the air from moving to the lungs, which decreases oxygen delivery to the body and brain.

Central sleep apnea occurs due to lack of brain signaling to respiratory muscles to breathe or due to paralysis of the breathing muscles themselves. Possible causes include structural defects of the brain, genetic disorders, brain tumor, trauma, infection, compression of the breathing centers in the brain stem, or due to injury to the upper part of the spinal cord that paralyzes the breathing muscles. A specific type of brain abnormality in which part of the brain is displaced into the spinal canal (called a Chiari malformation) can put pressure on the breathing centers in the brain and result in central apneas. In addition, central sleep apnea frequently occurs at high altitude due to the decreased oxygen content in the air. Infants also frequently have some degree of central sleep apnea that typically improves and resolves as they get older and their brain matures. Occasionally, heart problems can result in an unstable breathing pattern and central sleep apnea. Finally, certain medications, such as opioids, can decrease the drive to breathe and result in central sleep apnea.

How common is sleep apnea?

Symptoms of obstructive sleep apnea are common, with an estimated 5%-10% of children experiencing frequent snoring[1]. A smaller but still substantial number of children, about 1%-4%, meet the definition of obstructive sleep apnea based on sleep study criteria[1]. This percentage means that sleep apnea is one of the most prevalent diseases in children, more common than either epilepsy or diabetes. Despite the common occurrence of OSA, both public awareness and health care provider awareness of the disease is relatively low. As a result, the diagnosis is unfortunately frequently delayed or missed.

How is sleep apnea diagnosed?

The diagnosis of sleep apnea is based on a comprehensive evaluation by your child's doctor. This evaluation includes a comprehensive history, physical examination, and frequently further testing, such as sleep study, airway endoscopy, or brain imaging.

Your doctor may ask about symptoms of sleep apnea, such as snoring, mouth breathing, pauses in breathing, restless sleep, excessive night sweating, neck hyperextension during sleep, morning headaches, daytime sleepiness, attention or concentration problems at school, or symptoms of hyperactivity. You will likely be asked if your child has a family history of sleep apnea or other sleep or breathing disorders. It may be helpful to have a video clip of your child's typical breathing pattern during sleep to show your doctor.

During the physical examination, your child's doctor will evaluate the airway for potential contributing factors to airway obstruction. The doctor will likely evaluate the size of the tonsils, adenoids (if using a special camera to look in the nose), dental crowdedness, the roof of the mouth, tongue size, and the shape of the throat and jaw. Occasionally, airway endoscopy (looking in the airway with a camera) is used to further assess airway size and to screen for lesions or tissue that may be blocking the airway. This procedure could be performed by an ear, nose, and throat (ENT) physician in the clinic under local anesthetics, but may need to be performed under anesthesia, especially for younger children.

Based on your doctor's evaluation, further testing with a sleep study may be needed to confirm the sleep apnea diagnosis and assess the severity of disease. The type (obstructive or central) and severity (mild, moderate, or severe) of sleep apnea will dictate which therapeutic interventions are needed for your child (see Chapter 3 for an explanation of sleep studies and Chapter 4 for a discussion of treatment options). If there is a concern that your child has central sleep apnea, your physician may order a brain magnetic resonance imaging (MRI) and other tests to evaluate for possible causes of the central apneas.

What problems can sleep apnea cause?

Sleep apnea will lead to difficulty in breathing and intermittent decrease in oxygen delivery to the brain and body. An apnea or hypopnea results in a momentary decrease in oxygen levels. When the body senses this decrease in oxygen levels, as a protective mechanism it signals the brain to stimulate breathing to resume (partial awakening that is so brief that the patient does not remember it). With this arousal, the patient is able to open the airway, and oxygen will begin flowing back to the brain and body. When the brain falls back to sleep, another apnea can occur. The cycle can repeat all night long. The more frequent these events, the more severe sleep apnea is. All of these brief awakenings cause disrupted sleep, which in turn results in symptoms during the day, such as sleepiness, inattention, concentration problems, hyperactivity (especially in young children), poor school performance, and in some patients, symptoms of fatigue, or even depression. In addition, frequent intermittent decreases in oxygen to the body and brain and the increased work of breathing may lead to poor growth, systemic hypertension (high blood pressure in the body), pulmonary artery hypertension (high blood pressure between the heart and lungs), and even sudden death. Sleep apnea may result in long-term effects that may not appear until adulthood, such as hypertension, heart attacks, irregular heartbeat, and even stroke.

The effects of sleep apnea on behavior and learning have been the subject of many research studies. One of the first and most striking studies was performed in New Orleans by renowned sleep researcher David Gozal in 1998[2]. Dr. Gozal visited public schools in New Orleans to study children who were in the bottom 10% of their first grade class rankings. He found that 18% (54/297) of these children had sleep-disordered breathing. Of those 54 children, 24 then underwent surgical removal of their tonsils as treatment. The remaining 30 children had no treatment. The subsequent results one year later were striking. Among the 24 children who underwent treatment, grades increased almost a full letter grade. Only two remained in the lowest 10th percentile a year later. In contrast, those children who had no treatment had no change in their grades on average.

Over the last 20 years, many other studies have been performed to assess the impact of sleep apnea on learning and behavior, as well as the effects of treatment. Recent findings from a randomized trial (children randomly assigned to receive treatment vs no treatment) of surgical treatment for sleep apnea in children continue to support the premise that treating sleep apnea can substantially improve behavior problems in children[3]. Behavioral problems can be seen with any severity of sleep apnea[4]. A recent study of over 1,000 school-age children found that those behavioral problems can then lead to cognitive problems, affecting intelligence, reasoning, and language ability[5].

The figure below illustrates the effect of sleep apnea on cognitive function in children. The data is from published work by Dr. Gozal and colleagues[6]. DAS stands for Differential Abilities Scale, a formal test of reasoning and intellectual abilities. As the chart shows, children with sleep apnea, especially moderate to severe sleep apnea, have lower cognitive function scores.

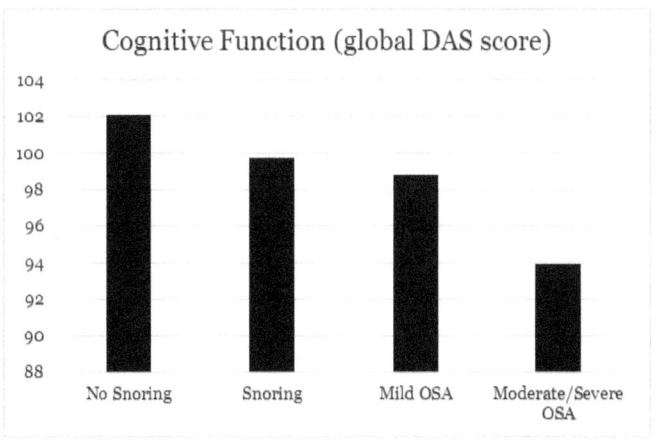

Beyond psychological testing and parent-reported behavioral problems, researchers have also examined effects on actual brain structure and function. Dr. Ann Halbower examined children with OSA and found significant IQ deficits compared to healthy children, but also changes in actual metabolism in multiple areas of the brain suggesting nerve cell injury[7]. Other studies have demonstrated decreased brain volume (size) in several regions of the brain of children with sleep apnea[8]. Studies have also shown that children with sleep apnea must exert more mental effort (neural recruitment) to perform at the same level as children without sleep apnea[9].

At the time of this writing, it is still unclear if snoring without sleep apnea (called primary snoring) can also cause behavioral and cognitive problems in children. This question remains an active area of research.

References

1. Lumeng JC, Chervin RD. Epidemiology of pediatric obstructive sleep apnea. Proc Am Thorac Soc. 2008 Feb 15;5(2):242-52.
2. Gozal D. Sleep-disordered breathing and school performance in children. Pediatrics. 1998 Sep;102(3 Pt 1):616-20.
3. Thomas NH, Xanthopoulos MS, Kim JY, et al. Effects of Adenotonsillectomy on Parent-Reported Behavior in Children With Obstructive Sleep Apnea. Sleep. 2017 Apr 1;40(4).
4. Smith DL, Gozal D, Hunter SJ, et al. Impact of sleep disordered breathing on behaviour among elementary school-aged children: a cross-sectional analysis of a large community-based sample. Eur Respir J. 2016 Dec;48(6):1631-1639.
5. Smith DL, Gozal D, Hunter SJ, et al. Parent-Reported Behavioral and Psychiatric Problems Mediate the Relationship between Sleep-Disordered Breathing and Cognitive Deficits in School-Aged Children. Front Neurol. 2017 Aug 11;8:410.
6. Hunter SJ, Gozal D, Smith DL, et al. Effect of Sleep-disordered Breathing Severity on Cognitive Performance Measures in a Large Community Cohort of Young School-aged Children. Am J Respir Crit Care Med. 2016 Sep 15;194(6):739-47.
7. Halbower AC, Degaonkar M, Barker PB, et al. Childhood obstructive sleep apnea associates with neuropsychological deficits and neuronal brain injury. PLoS Med. 2006 Aug;3(8):e301.
8. Philby MF, Macey PM, Ma RA, et al. Reduced

Regional Grey Matter Volumes in Pediatric Obstructive Sleep Apnea. Sci Rep. 2017 Mar 17;7:44566.

9. Kheirandish-Gozal L, Yoder K, Kulkarni R. Preliminary functional MRI neural correlates of executive functioning and empathy in children with obstructive sleep apnea. Sleep. 2014 Mar 1;37(3):587-92.

3

SLEEP STUDIES
Teresa J. Schneider, RPSGT

What is a sleep study?

A sleep study is a specialized test that analyzes a person's sleep. Recordings are made of brainwaves, eye movements, oxygen levels, carbon dioxide levels, heartbeat, airflow, breathing effort, and limb (leg) movements. This test helps the doctor know what is happening with the brain and breathing while the patient is asleep. A sleep study is performed during the night when the patient normally sleeps, and is called a polysomnogram.

This is what the sleep study looks like:

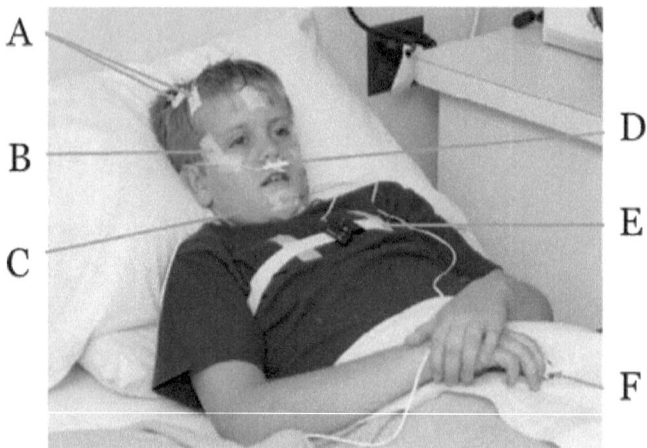

A: EEG sensors that monitor brain waves show when the patient is awake or asleep, and show what stage of sleep the patient is in.

B: Monitoring eye movements helps us to know when the patient is awake, asleep, or dreaming.

C: Chin muscle tone also shows when the patient is awake, asleep, or dreaming.

D: Nasal cannula and thermistor are sensors that monitor airflow and breathing.

E: Elastic belts measure chest and abdominal movements to assess breathing effort.

F: A pulse oximeter measures oxygen levels.

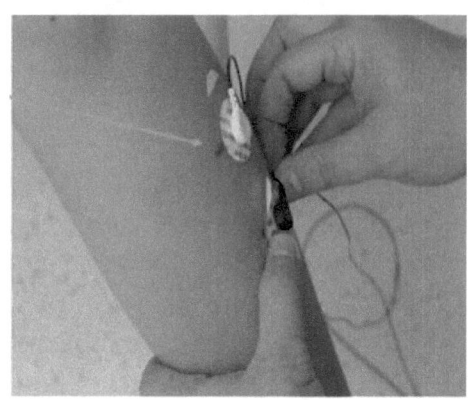

Sensors monitor leg movements during sleep

Who needs a sleep study?

Your child's doctor may order a sleep study if he or she is concerned that your child has a breathing disorder during sleep or frequent limb movements disrupting sleep, as part of an evaluation for narcolepsy, or to adjust CPAP settings. Symptoms of sleep apnea include snoring, gasping, snorting, night sweats, bedwetting, retractions, or paradoxical breathing (seesaw motion of chest and belly during sleep). Some children have other medical conditions that put them at increased risk for sleep apnea, such as Down syndrome, and may require a sleep study even if they do not exhibit any sleep symptoms at all. In addition, frequent leg movements, awakenings, and unrefreshing sleep may indicate a limb movement disorder during sleep that can be diagnosed on a sleep study. Finally, some symptoms that indicate the need for a sleep study can occur while the child is awake.

These symptoms include irritability, hyperactivity, sleepiness, and inattention. Specific breathing-related and non-breathing related reasons why your doctor may order a sleep study are listed in the tables below.

Breathing-related situations that may indicate the need to obtain a sleep study in children.

• Clinical concern for obstructive sleep apnea or other breathing disorders during sleep
• In children who have mild sleep apnea and undergo surgical treatment (T&A), but continue to have symptoms after surgery
• After T&A for all children with moderate/severe obstructive sleep apnea before surgery
• After T&A for all children with obesity, craniofacial abnormalities, Down syndrome, Prader-Willi syndrome, or other disorders that have lower surgical cure rates
• Adjusting CPAP pressures
• After treatment with rapid maxillary expander
• Oral appliance therapy
• Before removing tracheostomy

Non-breathing related reasons to obtain a sleep study in children.

• Clinical concern for periodic limb movement disorder (PLMD)
• Frequent parasomnias, seizures, or bedwetting
• Concern for narcolepsy or hypersomnia

What questions can a sleep study answer?

A sleep study can tell the doctor many things about your child's sleep. It can indicate whether the sleep patterns are normal, how much time it takes for your child to fall asleep, how long it takes your child to start to dream, whether the breathing patterns are normal or show pauses in breathing, how stable the oxygen and carbon dioxide levels are, and whether there are limb movements. The sleep study will also indicate how often breathing problems or limb movements occur and whether they cause your child's sleep to be disturbed.

In summary, a sleep study can help answer the following questions:

- Is sleep apnea or another breathing disorder present during sleep?
- Are excessive limb movements (PLMD) causing disrupted sleep?
- Is a given therapy (such as CPAP, maxillary expander, oral appliance, positional therapy) effective for treating the child's

sleep apnea?

- Is it safe to remove a child's tracheostomy?
- Are strange awakenings at night due to parasomnia (such as sleep terror)?
- Does a child have narcolepsy or other disorder of hypersomnia (if overnight sleep study is performed with next day nap test, called an MSLT)?

On the other hand, it is important to know which questions a sleep study cannot answer. A sleep study cannot always identify the problem with your child's sleep. For example, many children have behavioral insomnia, which is difficulty falling asleep or staying asleep because of the habits and behaviors that they have learned over time. Other children have restless legs syndrome (RLS), which is a creepy-crawly sensation in the legs that makes it difficult to fall asleep; this is a diagnosis made based on the history (clinical story/symptoms) provided by the patient. Still other children have sleep difficulties because their internal body clock (called circadian rhythm) is misaligned with the times when they ought to be awake or asleep. A sleep study performed in a child with these disorders may be completely normal, but that does not mean they don't have a sleep disorder. On the contrary, these disorders can and should be readily diagnosed based on the history alone. Therefore, parents should not feel disappointed if a child's provider does not feel that a sleep study is needed. The most important sleep test your child can have is an astute sleep provider listening closely to history provided by parent and child.

How do I prepare my child for a sleep study?

There are just a few preparation instructions for a sleep study. Your child should be bathed the day of the study and have no lotions or ointments put on the skin. (This will help our sensors to stay on.) Your child's hair should be freshly washed and have no products put in it. If your child is over the age of 3, do not have them nap during the day of the study. If your child is under 3, try to limit napping during the day of the study to 1 hour or less. There should be no caffeine use the day of the study; this includes caffeine-containing foods such as chocolate. Sometimes the doctor ordering the sleep study will stop some medications for a period of time before the sleep study. Several pediatric sleep centers have developed excellent instructional videos that can help to prepare your child for what to expect. One such video, produced at Children's Mercy Hospital, is available for viewing here:

https://www.childrensmercy.org/Clinics_and_Ser vices/Clinics_and_Departments/Sleep_Disorders_ Program/

While most children tolerate a sleep study without much of a problem, some do not. Sometimes knowing if a child will tolerate a sleep study can be difficult to predict, but you as the parent know your child best and probably will be able to judge your child's likelihood of successfully completing the sleep study. If you are unsure or feel that your child will find the test challenging, request a tour of the sleep lab during the day, well before the scheduled sleep study. Planning ahead like this allows the opportunity for your child to see the sensors, staff, and facility spaces. For many children, this helps to alleviate fears.

For those children who continue to struggle, many pediatric sleep centers offer "desensitization" appointments. Desensitization simply means working with providers (sometimes sleep techs, sometimes psychologists) to gradually expose the child to the sensors for increasing amounts of time until the child is able to tolerate them long enough to complete the sleep study. Many times, desensitization involves a combination of in-person appointments with a member of the sleep lab team, as well as home practice with a sleep study "training kit." The kit includes materials that mimic the sensors that will be used the night of the sleep study (such as paper tape to imitate pulse oximeter, stickers for leads on the face, neck, and legs, gauze to mimic chest/belly belts and to wrap the head, and a nasal cannula). Parents will continue to practice with the child with a goal of the child being able to fall asleep with the "sensors" in place. With continued practice, almost all children, even those with special needs or sensory issues, are able to successfully complete a sleep study.

How should I pack for the sleep study?

Sleep studies are performed on an outpatient basis. You should pack as if you were going to a hotel. Bring any medications that you will need to give to your child during the course of the study. You will also need to bring things like pajamas, diapers, wipes, and formula if you will need them. We encourage you to bring your child's favorite pillow or stuffed animal to have something from home. You may also bring a favorite DVD to play that will help distract your child during the set up procedure.

How will my child be able to sleep with all of the equipment on?

The sleep study is a very unusual condition for sleep. The night of sleep in the lab will probably not be as good as it might be at home. In fact, studies have been done where children undergo sleep studies on consecutive nights, and they tend to sleep better on the second night compared to the first (this is called a "first night effect"). In contrast, breathing tends to be similar night to night (except if a child is sick with a cold or other illness). Therefore, even if your child doesn't sleep well the night of her sleep study, she will almost certainly sleep enough for us to determine whether she has a breathing problem during sleep.

How is the sleep study interpreted?

Once the sleep study is completed, there is still much work to be done. The study first needs to be scored. During scoring, a sleep technologist will look through each page, or "epoch," of the sleep recording (which equals 30 seconds of recording time) and assign a sleep stage. Then the technologist will review the recording again to mark breathing events and limb movements. The technologist will also go through the heartbeat tracings and look for anything abnormal (arrhythmias). Once the record is scored, the sleep physician will review the entire recording and look at the results of the scoring in order to formulate a final interpretation. This interpretation, along with a summary of all of the measurements performed during the sleep study, are combined into a final sleep study report.

A snapshot view of the entire sleep study can also be seen by looking at the hypnogram. The hypnogram displays much of the information collected during a sleep study in a summary illustration, typically incorporating sleep stages, respiratory events, body position, limb movements, oxygen saturations, CO_2 levels, respiratory rate, and heart rate, among other measures. An example hypnogram is seen below.

Example Hypnogram.

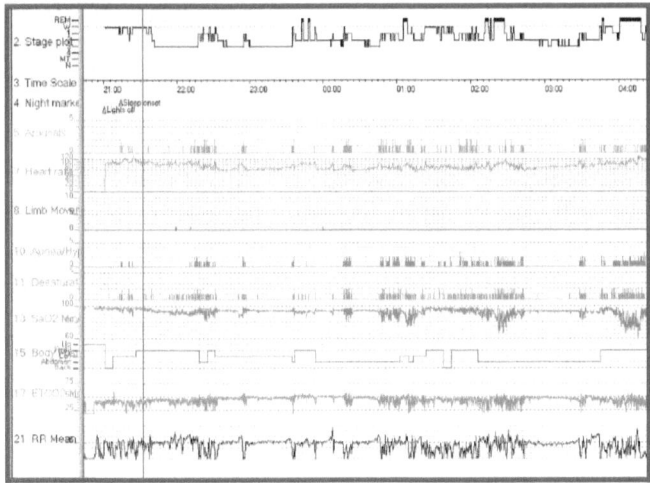

What do all the numbers on the report mean?

If you look at your child's sleep study report, chances are you are overwhelmed by the amount of information and are wondering what all of those numbers mean. In general, the numbers can be divided into one of a few general measures, which include sleep staging and architecture, breathing, limb movements, and video clips.

At its most basic level, a sleep study measures sleep, which can be summarized in numbers that describe the sleep architecture. In fact, as a parent you are likely very interested in exactly how much "deep sleep" or "dream sleep" your child achieved during his sleep study. One of the first numbers the report will give is the sleep efficiency. This is the percentage of the recording time the patient was actually asleep during the night. Sleep efficiency can be an indicator of how disturbed a patient's sleep is, and is many times lower when a child has a sleep disorder such as sleep apnea or even narcolepsy. Sleep latency is reported in minutes and tells how long it took the patient to fall asleep once the actual test was started. Sleep comes in different stages. Each night the sleep stages cycle, and each sleep stage represents a percentage of the night. The report will show how much the patient slept in each sleep stage.

Another measure of sleep architecture is arousals, or brief awakenings. The report will also give a total number of arousals and an arousal index. An arousal means any time the patient's sleep became lighter or they woke up completely. The arousal index indicates how many arousals they had per each hour of sleep.

Breathing is characterized in several ways. Each pause (apnea) and shallow breath (hypopnea) is tabulated and the total number of these events per hour of sleep is called the apnea-hypopnea index, or AHI. The AHI is our current "measuring stick" for sleep apnea, and is important for making the diagnosis and tracking severity. We further break these events down into those respiratory events that are caused by airway obstruction (obstructive AHI, or OAHI), and those that are not due to obstruction (central AHI, or CAHI). Since respiratory events can be more common while sleeping on the back (supine), the report will also give the supine AHI and the non-supine AHI. This measure tells us whether the sleep apnea is worse while the patient is supine. Likewise, REM (dream) sleep is also a common time to see more frequent breathing events, so the report may also give a REM and non-REM AHI.

Besides apneas and hypopneas, important breathing parameters include oxygen and carbon dioxide (CO_2) levels throughout the night. Normally, we breathe in oxygen, our body uses it, and CO_2 is exhaled as a waste product. However, oxygen and CO_2 levels can be abnormal in several different diseases. For example, sleep apnea can cause airway obstruction, which can result in low oxygen levels (because oxygen can't get in) as well as high CO_2 levels (because CO_2 can't get out). In addition, asthma or other lung diseases can cause low oxygen levels during sleep. Significantly low oxygen levels are called hypoxemia, and high CO_2 levels are called hypoventilation.

Limb movements sometimes disrupt sleep and are tabulated throughout the night. Limb movements that come in groups are called periodic limb movements (PLMs), and the number of these per hour is called the periodic limb movement index (PLMI). Children with frequent PLMs and clinically disrupted sleep may have periodic limb movement disorder (PLMD).

Finally, a review of video clips of sleep during the night can be extremely helpful. For instance, parasomnias that occur during the night, such as sleep terrors, may be identified and diagnosed. In addition, watching the child's work of breathing is essential. Children who appear to be working hard to breathe (with retractions, paradoxical breathing, mouth breathing, and neck hyperextension) are likely have significant sleep apnea.

Key measures from a sleep study.

Sleep efficiency	The percentage of time spent in bed when the child is actually asleep.
Sleep latency	The time it takes for the child to fall asleep from lights out.
REM latency	The time it takes for the child to achieve first REM sleep.
N1 N2 N3 R	The percentage of sleep time spent in each sleep stage. N1 and N2 are "light sleep," N3 is "deep sleep," and R is REM or "dream sleep."
Arousal index	The number of arousals (ranging from 3 seconds to full awakening) per hour of sleep.
AHI	The number of pauses (apneas) and shallow breaths (hypopneas) per hour of sleep.
Periodic limb movement index	The number of limb movements that come in groups (periodic) per hour of sleep.
Video clips	Description of observed breathing (snoring, etc.) and any clinical events (such as parasomnia).

4

TREATING SLEEP APNEA
David G. Ingram, MD

What are the treatment options?

When sleep apnea was first recognized and diagnosed, the only treatment option was a surgically created hole in the neck, called a tracheostomy, to bypass the upper airway obstruction. Thankfully, due to technological advancements and research efforts, clinicians now have many tools at their disposal when caring for children with sleep apnea. Even with increasing options, though, there is no "cookie cutter" approach that is right for every child. Instead, the options are like a treatment menu. We select the items from the menu that best suit the particular patient we are seeing. In other words, while one particular child may need only a single treatment type, another child may require a combination or sequence of treatments for best results. The differences in treatment plans are usually due to sleep apnea type (obstructive or central), severity (mild, moderate, severe), or the child's other underlying health problems, physical exam findings, and the way families and health care providers weigh risks and benefits.

In general, the sleep apnea treatment menu includes surgery (such as removing the tonsils and adenoids), positive airway pressure (CPAP is the most common), medications, orthodontics, oxygen, weight management, positioning, and myofunctional therapy (exercises to strengthen muscles in the mouth and throat). In this chapter, we will explain the current common treatment approaches, as well as emerging new therapies that researchers are testing.

Do we have to treat sleep apnea or will my child grow out of it?

Before we look at the different treatment options for sleep apnea, we should first step back and ask the most basic question: Does sleep apnea really require treatment at all? First, we must know the risks of untreated sleep apnea versus the risks of treatment.

As outlined in Chapter 2, untreated sleep apnea

may contribute to a vast array of health problems, including problems with school performance, attention and learning, behavior, growth, and heart disease. Even so, nearly every treatment has potential downsides: surgery and anesthesia can have complications, medications may have side effects, and CPAP may cause a nightly battle of wills between child and parent.

While the overwhelming opinion has been that the benefits of treatment outweigh the risks, researchers only very recently addressed this question scientifically. In 2013, a landmark research study (the Childhood Adenotonsillectomy Trial, or CHAT[1]) randomized (randomly assigned) children with diagnosed obstructive sleep apnea to either be treated (by surgical removal of the tonsils and adenoids) or not (watchful waiting). After a period of 7 months, children who had undergone treatment were found to have improved behavior, quality of life, sleep study findings, and some measures of cognitive function (nonverbal reasoning, fine motor skills, and selective attention)[2].

The below chart is based on data from the CHAT study discussed above and demonstrates greater improvements in children who underwent T&A compared to watchful waiting: improvements are noted in behavior (Conners' and BRIEF scores), symptoms of sleep apnea (PSQ-SRBD scale), overall quality of life (PedsQL), and sleep study findings (AHI).

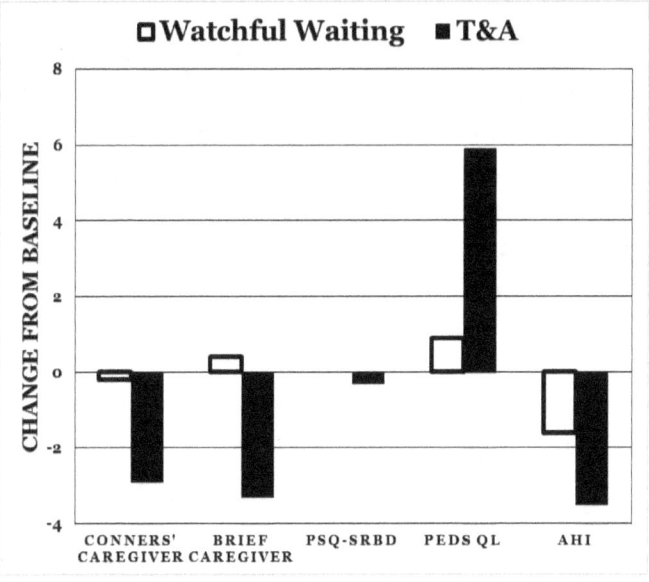

Researchers then examined the outcomes of those children who were in the "watchful waiting" group and did not undergo surgery[3]. Interestingly, they found that almost one-half (42%) of those children no longer demonstrated sleep apnea on their sleep studies after 7 months. Those children with mild sleep apnea (AHI<5/hr) and less central obesity (normal waist circumference) were most likely to have spontaneous resolution of their sleep apnea. The researchers speculated that spontaneous reduction in tonsil size or airway growth over time could explain the improvement. In contrast to many children having spontaneous improvement on their sleep studies, only 15% of children had any substantial improvement in their caregiver-reported sleep apnea symptoms (sleepiness, snoring, and behavior problems). Those children with the mildest symptoms were more likely to have their symptoms resolve. Taken together, the results showed that watchful waiting may be a reasonable option for children with few symptoms, minimal snoring, no obesity, and only mild sleep apnea on their sleep study.

One possible explanation for the discrepancy in a "spontaneously normalized" sleep study versus continued problematic symptoms is that the AHI measure from sleep studies may not capture more subtle signs of upper airway obstruction. This possibility was illustrated in a study where the children who had spontaneous resolution of their sleep apnea (according to AHI) were compared to those who had resolution after surgery. The researchers found that those who had spontaneous resolution continued to have thoraco-abdominal asynchrony (also known as paradoxical breathing), whereas those who underwent surgery did not[4]. Paradoxical breathing is a sign of upper airway obstruction seen during sleep studies. The researchers found that children who had continued paradoxical respirations had lower quality of life compared to those that did not have paradoxical respirations.

Overall, while a small subset of children may "outgrow" their sleep apnea, these children are typically mildly affected in the first place. If you are taking your child to a sleep provider or for a sleep study, you have probably noticed symptoms that make you concerned that your child is having significant sleep or behavioral problems. Therefore, "watchful waiting" may not be appropriate, because moderate and severe symptoms are unlikely to resolve without treatment. Additionally, several treatment options are available for mild sleep apnea beyond or instead of surgery (we'll discuss them below). In any case, if you choose a strategy of "watchful waiting," it's important to follow up with your doctor so that you do not miss an opportunity to improve the health of your child.

Most adults I know who have been diagnosed with sleep apnea have to use a CPAP machine. Will my child have to wear one of those?

Positive airway pressure, usually continuous positive airway pressure (CPAP), is the treatment most often used for obstructive sleep apnea in adults. For children, because their airway obstruction may be due to enlarged tonsils and adenoids, surgery is usually considered first. Even so, many children use and benefit from CPAP for sleep apnea. CPAP is most often used in children who have moderate or severe obstructive sleep apnea but do not appear to have enlarged tonsils or adenoids or other obvious surgical sites of obstruction.

In addition, CPAP may be used if a child has already had tonsils and adenoids removed but still has moderate or severe obstructive sleep apnea (OSA) after surgery. Some children who do have enlarged tonsils and adenoids may have other health problems that place them at increased risk for complications during or after surgery and so are placed on CPAP instead. Likewise, some children with very severe obstructive sleep apnea may be set up on CPAP ahead of surgery for a smoother recovery. Finally, CPAP is an option for those families who have a strong desire for a non-surgical treatment option for their child's sleep apnea. In summary, while CPAP is definitely on the treatment menu and works well to treat sleep apnea, it is typically employed in certain clinical situations rather than as a standard first-line treatment as it is in adults. See Chapter 6 for more information about CPAP.

What surgeries can treat sleep apnea?

While this topic will be covered in detail in Chapter 5, we will provide an overview of possible surgeries for obstructive sleep apnea.

By far, the most common treatment for obstructive sleep apnea in children is adenotonsillectomy (T&A), surgical removal of the tonsils and adenoids. In fact, T&A is generally considered first-line therapy for children older than 2 years who have enlarged tonsils and adenoids on exam. The adenoids are positioned in the back of the nasal airway, so cannot be seen on physical exam without transnasal laryngoscopy (sticking a camera in the nose). Therefore, most sleep providers who are not ear, nose and throat physicians (ENTs) will not be able to tell you if the adenoids are contributing to the obstruction; this will only be revealed during surgery when they are visualized directly. In contrast, the tonsils can be seen by looking in the back of the throat during a routine physical exam. Potential complications of surgery include throat pain, bleeding, breathing problems, and infection.

T&A is generally effective. In the CHAT study discussed above, 79% of children had a normal sleep study after surgery. However, only healthy children without significant medical problems were included in that study. Children with other health problems, such as children with Down syndrome or obesity, have lower rates of surgical success. For example, in a review of studies which included 1,079 children who underwent T&A, uncomplicated patients had a cure rate of 73%, compared to 38% cure rate in complicated patients (obese children, severe sleep apnea, or young age)[5]. Likewise, a recent study of T&A in children with Down syndrome demonstrated that about half had continued moderate to severe sleep apnea even after surgery[6].

Certain patient groups have lower cure rates most

likely because they have multiple reasons for airway obstruction. For example, children with Down syndrome often have enlarged tonsils and adenoids, low muscle tone, large tongues, and different facial and airway structures, any of which can contribute to obstructive sleep apnea. While removing the tonsils and adenoids almost always helps (and is still usually the first step in treatment), it addresses only one of those reasons for obstruction, and so it is less likely to result in total cure compared to a surgery in a generally healthy child.

Besides removing tonsils and adenoids (T&A), other surgeries have been developed that may be helpful for obstructive sleep apnea in children. Some children, especially those with Down syndrome, may have significant airway obstruction if the back of the tongue falls into the airway. Therefore, surgery to remove tissue from the back half of the tongue, called base of tongue reduction surgery, can sometimes be helpful. Similarly, another set of tonsils sit behind the tongue, and these "tongue tonsils" (called lingual tonsils) can be removed (lingual tonsillectomy) if they are creating obstruction. Other children, especially younger children and infants, may have soft floppy tissue above the vocal cords that can cause obstruction (called laryngomalacia), and this tissue can be surgically trimmed down in a procedure called supraglottoplasty. Infants may also have airway obstruction due to a small lower jaw (called micrognathia), which occurs most commonly with a disorder called Pierre Robin sequence. Surgeons can move the lower jaw forward by cutting the bone and placing a small metal rod (called a distractor) that slowly stretches the jaw apart (mandibular distraction osteogenesis). A common adult procedure is called a UPPP (which stands for uvulopalatopharyngoplasty), in which soft tissue is surgically removed from the back of the throat. Combining the UPPP with T&A is rarely done in children at this time. Tracheostomy, which used to be the only treatment for sleep apnea in children, is now used only as a last resort in children who have very severe sleep apnea that cannot be managed otherwise.

Can medications help?

Children with obstructive sleep apnea tend to have inflammation in the upper airway. While the exact cause is not known, theories include tissue damage and inflammation from snoring vibrations and repetitive pressure swings, or inflammation from free radicals produced by repeated fluctuations in oxygen levels. In addition, chronic nasal congestion, for example due to seasonal allergies, can contribute to nasal airway obstruction and worsen sleep apnea.

It is therefore unsurprising that researchers have found that some anti-inflammatory medications can be effective for treating mild cases of obstructive sleep apnea. Specifically, nasal steroids (such as fluticasone) and oral leukotriene inhibitors (such as montelukast) are both medications that are typically used for seasonal allergies, but may be also effective for sleep apnea in children. This therapy was pioneered and further developed by Dr. Gozal and colleagues. They recently reviewed over 750 of their patients who had been placed on a combination of nasal steroids and oral montelukast for mild OSA (AHI 1-5/hr). They found that over 80% had some improvement and 62% were "cured" (defined by normal follow-up sleep study)[7]. Currently, these medications are most commonly used in children who have mild OSA and a non-surgical treatment option is preferred, or in children who have mild OSA after having T&A.

What other treatments may be helpful?

Obesity is a major contributor to sleep apnea in children, likely due to fat deposited in the airway and tongue. In one study, obese children had a 4-5 times increased risk of having sleep apnea compared to non-obese children[8]. Therefore, working on fitness and nutrition to optimize weight should be on the treatment menu for all obese children with sleep apnea.

During sleep, the airway tends to be more collapsible when people lie on their back, likely due to the effects of gravity. As a result, sleep apnea tends to be worse when children sleep on their back compared to their side or stomach. In some children, sleep apnea occurs almost exclusively when they are on their back, and in these cases positional therapy may be helpful. Your provider may prescribe a device that is worn at night and is specifically designed to help keep people from sleeping on their back.

Some children have a high-arched palate (roof of the mouth). The palate in the mouth also makes up the bottom of the airway in the nose. Consequently, high-arched palate can decrease the space for air to flow in the nose (increase nasal resistance to airflow) and contribute to obstructive sleep apnea. For this reason, children with a high-arched palate can benefit from a rapid maxillary expander (RME). An RME is an orthodontic device that can slowly expand the palate. It is typically in place for about 3 to 6 months, and can be an effective treatment for obstructive sleep apnea.

Another way to increase the size of the upper airway without surgery or CPAP is by moving the lower jaw forward. Dental sleep specialists can make a mandibular advancement device (also called oral appliance) that is worn at night and pushes the lower jaw forward compared to the upper jaw. These devices are much more commonly used in adult patients with obstructive sleep apnea, but are beginning to be tested and used in children[9]. If this treatment option is pursued, it is important to seek a qualified and credentialed sleep dentist. A list of dentists that are certified by the

American Board of Dental Sleep Medicine (ABDSM) can be found at: http://www.aadsm.org/FindADentist.aspx.

One important contributing factor to obstructive sleep apnea is upper airway muscle tone. Because the dilator muscles help keep the upper airway open and prevent obstruction, researchers have investigated various exercises to help strengthen those muscles. Myofunctional therapy (also called myofascial reeducation, oromyofacial therapy, or orofacial myology) is a set of muscle exercises aimed at retraining the muscles of the tongue and upper airway to improve tone and nasal airflow. In fact, several studies have now demonstrated myofunctional therapy to be effective at decreasing the severity of obstructive sleep apnea in children, and is typically used in combination with other treatment modalities (such as T&A or RME)[10]. A list of therapists that have been certified by the International Association of Orofacial Myology (IAOM) can be found at: http://iaom.com/.

Typically, the airway is most prone to collapse at the end of expiration. Therefore, a device has been developed that acts as a one-way valve for the nose, providing no resistance to inhalation in the nose, but increased resistance during expiration. The goal is to increase pressure in the airway during expiration to prevent the airway collapse. This device is referred to as a nasal expiratory positive pressure device (NEPAP). NEPAP devices have been tested in and used in adults for some time, and are just starting to be trialed in children. One small pilot study in children with OSA by researchers in Philadelphia did demonstrate that using this device resulted in significant improvements compared to a placebo (mock) device; older children and those with less elevation in their CO_2 levels during sleep had better responses to the device[11].

All of the treatments discussed above are for obstructive sleep apnea (OSA), but my child has been diagnosed with central sleep apnea (CSA). What can be done for CSA?

There are two basic reasons why a pause in breathing may occur during sleep. First, the airway can collapse, and although the child will still be attempting to breathe (moving the chest and belly) he cannot move air through the collapsed airway; this is obstructive apnea. The second reason that a child can have a pause in breathing is if there is a problem in the signal traveling from the brain to the|body to tell it when to take a breath. There can be several different reasons for central apneas to occur in children, so it is important that a sleep provider assess for those underlying causes, such as neurological problems that can affect breathing centers in the brain.

In terms of treatment, there are several options. The first important step is making sure that any underlying conditions contributing to the central apnea are treated. As an example, some children have a structural brain abnormality where part of the brain is displaced into the spinal canal (called a Chiari malformation). This displacement can put pressure on the breathing centers in the brain and result in central apneas. A Chiari malformation is diagnosed by performing an MRI of the brain, and surgery can be performed to correct Chiari malformation, potentially curing the central sleep apnea.

If central sleep apnea still is problematic despite addressing potential underlying causes, other therapies may be required. While CPAP is often used for OSA, there are a variety of modes of positive airway pressure beyond CPAP. Specifically, while CPAP provides a constant level of pressure, there are devices that provide a higher pressure during inspiration and lower pressure during expiration. One such mode is called a bi-level positive airway pressure (BPAP ST) because there are two levels of pressure. BPAP ST can be used to treat central sleep apnea as long as a backup rate is used (denoted by the "ST" in the name, whereby the machine will provide a breath if it senses a pause in breathing). BPAP without a backup rate may actually worsen central apneas, so the backup rate is very important. Another more advanced mode is called adaptive servo-ventilation (ASV). Just like BPAP ST, ASV provides a higher pressure during inspiration and a lower pressure during expiration as well as a backup rate. The additional feature that ASV provides is that the machine automatically changes the inspiratory pressure over time throughout the night depending on the respiratory pattern. These different modes of positive airway pressure are discussed further in Chapter 6.

One of the most commonly used therapies for CSA in children, especially infants, is simply supplemental oxygen during sleep. Oxygen can stabilize the pattern of breathing and prevent the oxygen desaturations associated with central apneas. Many infants with central sleep apnea may be treated with oxygen temporarily and eventually grow out of their apnea so they no longer need treatment[12].

Finally, certain medications can also be effective for central sleep apnea. Acetazolamide is a medication that works by causing a mild buildup of acid in the body (acidosis); this acidosis stimulates the drive to breathe, which in turn decreases central apneas. Another medication that works in a different manner but can also stimulate breathing and decrease central apneas is called theophylline. Both of these medications have side effects. Therefore, close monitoring with your physician is critically important.

Are there any new treatments on the horizon?

In fact, there is an exciting new surgical treatment, called hypoglossal nerve stimulation, currently under investigation by researchers. The hypoglossal nerve controls the tongue muscles and several other muscles of the upper airway. The hypoglossal nerve stimulator is a device that is surgically implanted and stimulates the hypoglossal nerve to keep the airway open during sleep. Patients turn the device on and off with a remote.

Currently, this device is only approved and available for patients who are older than 21 years. However, researchers in Boston implanted the first device in a 14-year-old child with Down syndrome and severe OSA who required tracheostomy despite previous T&A in April 2015; the child's sleep apnea was almost completely resolved (AHI decreased from 48/hr to 3/hr), and the child was able to have the tracheostomy removed five months after implantation of the nerve stimulator[13].

At the time of writing this book, a larger trial testing the effectiveness of hypoglossal nerve stimulation in children with Down syndrome was ongoing with results pending. Clearly, hypoglossal nerve stimulation has potential to be on the OSA treatment menu for children in the near future.

References

1. Marcus CL, et al. A randomized trial of adenotonsillectomy for childhood sleep apnea. N Engl J Med. 2013 Jun 20;368(25):2366-76.
2. Taylor HG, et al. Cognitive effects of adenotonsillectomy for obstructive sleep apnea. Pediatrics. 2016 Aug;138(2): e20154458.
3. Chervin RD, et al. Prognosis for Spontaneous Resolution of OSA in Children. Chest. 2015 Nov;148(5):1204-1213.
4. Liu X, et al. Adenotonsillectomy for childhood obstructive sleep apnoea reduces thoraco-abdominal asynchrony but spontaneous apnoea-hypopnoea index normalisation does not. Eur Respir J. 2017 Jan 25;49(1). pii: 1601177.
5. Friedman M, et al. Updated systematic review of tonsillectomy and adenoidectomy for treatment of pediatric obstructive sleep apnea/hypopnea syndrome. Otolaryngol Head Neck Surg. 2009 Jun;140(6):800-8.
6. Ingram DG, et al. Success of Tonsillectomy for Obstructive Sleep Apnea in Children With Down Syndrome. J Clin Sleep Med. 2017 Aug 15;13(8):975-980.
7. Kheirandish-Gozal L, et al. Antiinflammatory therapy outcomes for mild OSA in children. Chest. 2014 Jul;146(1):88-95.
8. Redline S, et al. Risk factors for sleep-disordered breathing in children. Associations with obesity, race, and respiratory problems. Am J Respir Crit Care Med. 1999 May;159(5 Pt 1):1527-32.
9. Nazarali N, et al. Mandibular advancement appliances for the treatment of paediatric obstructive sleep apnea: a systematic review. Eur

J Orthod. 2015 Dec;37(6):618-26.

10. Camacho M, et al. Myofunctional Therapy to Treat Obstructive Sleep Apnea: A Systematic Review and Meta-analysis. Sleep. 2015 May 1;38(5):669-75.

11. Kureshi SA, et al. Pilot study of nasal expiratory positive airway pressure devices for the treatment of childhood obstructive sleep apnea syndrome. J Clin Sleep Med. 2014 Jun 15;10(6):663-9.

12. Deschamp A & Daftary A. A Newborn Infant With Oxygen Desaturation During Sleep. Chest. 2017 Jan;151(1):e17-e20.

13. Diercks GR, et al. Hypoglossal Nerve Stimulator Implantation in an Adolescent With Down Syndrome and Sleep Apnea. Pediatrics. 2016 May;137(5). pii: e20153663.

5

SURGERY FOR SLEEP APNEA
Jill M. Arganbright, MD
Hayat Adib, MD

What are tonsils?

Tonsils are soft tissue collections made up of lymphoid tissue, part of the immune system. They are positioned in the back of the throat. Some children's tonsils are small and some are so enlarged that they are touching one another, which we call "kissing tonsils." We use a specific grading system to determine how large the tonsils are. The grading system is as follows:

- Grade 0: Tonsils absent, surgically removed.
- Grade 1: Hidden behind tonsillar pillars.
- Grade 2: Extend to pillars.
- Grade 3: Visible beyond pillars.

- Grade 4: Reach midline, these are called kissing tonsils.

Sometimes, when tonsils are enlarged they can obstruct part of the back of the throat while the child is sleeping, causing obstructive breathing at night.

Below is a picture obtained during surgery of a patient's tonsils.

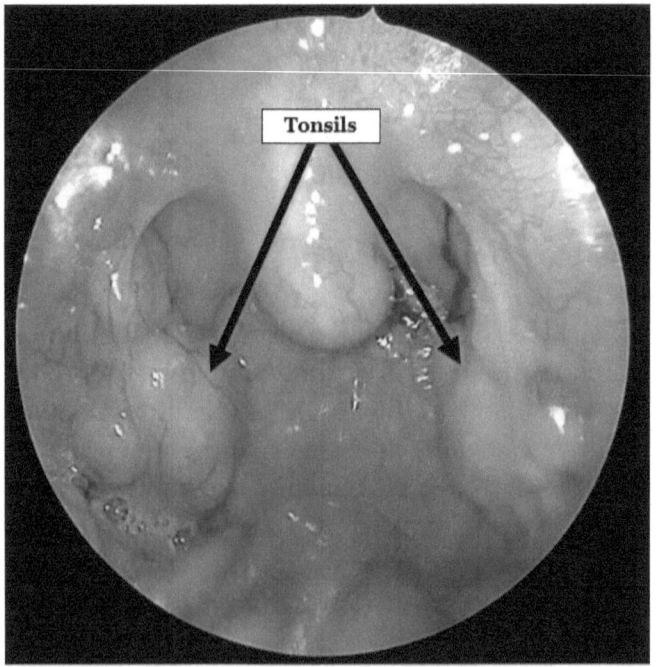

What are adenoids?

Adenoids are a soft tissue collection positioned in

the very back of the nose, in an anatomic region called the nasopharynx. They are made up of lymphoid tissue, similar to the tonsils. When the adenoids are enlarged, they can make breathing through the nose difficult. Because the adenoids are in the very back of the nose, they are not visible "just by looking" in the nose. The adenoids require a scope placed into the nostril and advanced to the very back of the nose to visualize. The adenoid tissue usually fades away, or "atrophies," in our adult years.

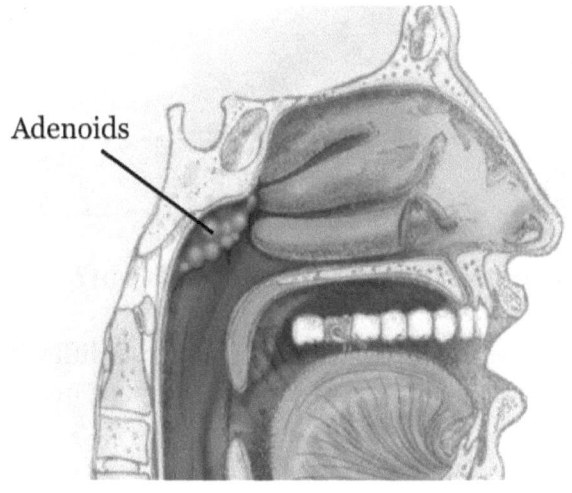

Although tonsils and adenoids are comprised of lymphoid tissue and considered part of the immune system, many studies have demonstrated that there are no negative effects on immune function after removing the tonsils and adenoids[1].

Below is a picture obtained during surgery of a child's adenoids.

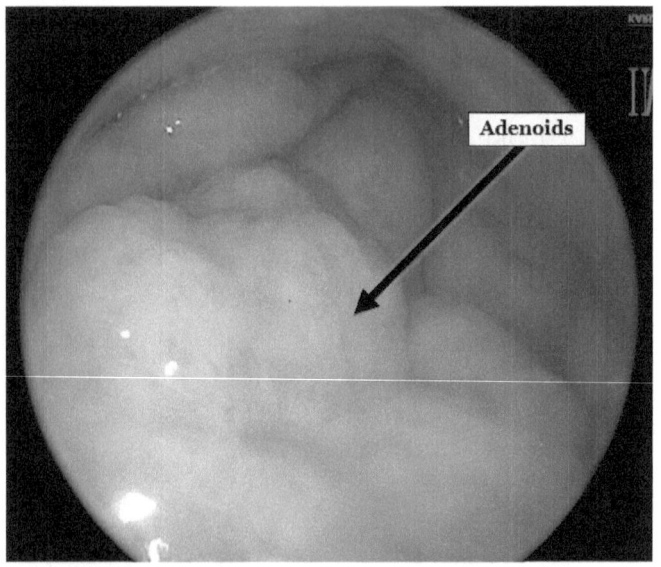

Why take the tonsils and adenoids out?

Enlarged tonsils and adenoids can cause difficulty breathing at night, which can lead to poor quality sleep.

For children 2 years of age or older who have a sleep study with obstructive sleep apnea, removal of the tonsils and adenoids is currently considered first-line surgical therapy.

In children who have not had a sleep study, the provider will look for certain signs and symptoms to suggest obstructive breathing at night; when a child has these signs and symptoms, it is called clinical "obstructive sleep-disordered breathing."

Signs to watch for during the night that may suggest sleep-disordered breathing:

- Loud nightly snoring (sometimes may sound as loud as a grown man's).
- Pauses in breathing or gasps for air, similar to sleep apnea.
- Restless sleep.
- Frequently waking up at night.
- Bedwetting at an older age or after a period of dryness.

If a child is getting poor sleep quality at night, this may cause various symptoms to carry over and affect the child during the day. Signs to watch for during the daytime that may suggest sleep-disordered breathing:

- Difficulty getting up in the morning.
- Not appearing to have gotten a good night's sleep.
- Needing extra naps during the day.
- Daytime hyperactivity.
- Headaches in the morning.

If these symptoms are present, a referral to an ear, nose, and throat provider to evaluate the size of tonsils and adenoids should be considered. If the patient has symptoms of sleep-disordered breathing AND large tonsils or adenoids are found on exam, the child may benefit from surgery; in most cases, removing the enlarged tonsils or adenoids will improve the symptoms of sleep-disordered breathing.

It is important to note that not all children with large tonsils have obstructive breathing at night. Therefore, if a patient has very large tonsils but no symptoms of sleep-disordered breathing, then the tonsils do not necessarily need to be removed.

What should I expect during and after my child's adenotonsillectomy?

The surgery for removing tonsils and adenoids is called adenotonsillectomy (abbreviated, T&A). This is a very common and safe operation. The surgery takes about 45 minutes, and requires general anesthesia. Typically, the throat will be sore for about 1-2 weeks after the surgery. Pain medications will be needed during the recovery period and the regimen will be discussed in detail with you by the surgeon. The child will need to stay the first week after surgery at home with a family member. The second week the child is generally able to return to school, although she will need a full two weeks off of heavy or rough activity, recess, gym class, and sports. It is important that children continue to drink liquids frequently (even if the child does not want to) throughout the recovery process to prevent dehydration. Of note, the tonsillectomy portion of the procedure is usually not recommended for children under 2 years old.

Will my child have to stay in the hospital overnight?

There are many factors that determine whether your child will need to stay overnight at the hospital or be released the same day as surgery. All children under 3 years old, those with severe obstructive sleep apnea, obesity, or with other specific medical conditions or syndromes will be asked to spend the night. These children are at higher risk for complications following surgery so are watched closely to ensure safe recovery immediately after surgery.

What are the possible complications of adenotonsillectomy?

Adenotonsillectomy is a very common and safe operation, although like other surgeries, is not without risks. The main risks of removing the tonsils are:

- Bleeding during surgery: rarely, severe bleeding occurs during the surgery and may require additional treatments or a longer hospital stay.
- Bleeding during healing: there is a 3% risk[2] of bleeding from the mouth where the tonsils

were removed during the first 2 weeks after surgery. These 2 weeks are the time frame that the wound from the tonsillectomy is healing; if a scab from the wound is dislodged too soon, bleeding can occur. If there is any bleeding after surgery, the child should be brought to the emergency room immediately!

The risk of removing the adenoids is very small:

- Adenoid regrowth: the adenoids can re-grow and need a second procedure to remove the additional adenoid tissue. This is rare and more commonly occurs in younger children having their adenoids removed. Regrowth is not usually significant enough to warrant repeat surgery. It is estimated that 0.5%-3% of patients would require a repeat adenoidectomy[3].
- Hypernasal speech: if this is present after adenoidectomy, you should let your surgeon know. Often, this is caused by the child having an abnormal alignment of the muscles in the soft palate.

Lastly, there is a risk that the adenotonsillectomy does not improve the sleep-disordered breathing. If symptoms do not resolve after the surgery, obtaining a sleep study is essential to accurately assess disease severity, and more surgery or other treatment may be needed in the future.

How well does adenotonsillectomy work for sleep apnea?

Generally speaking, the adenotonsillectomy procedure is effective for children with obstructive sleep apnea or sleep-disordered breathing. Many factors contribute to the overall likelihood of improvement with surgery alone. Children with Down syndrome have about a 50% risk of still having moderate to severe disease even after the adenotonsillectomy[4]. Children who are obese are also at a high risk of surgery not completely fixing the symptoms. The surgeon will specifically discuss the expected outcome, risks, benefits, and alternatives when explaining the procedure.

Do you have to take both the tonsils and adenoids out, or just one or the other?

The surgeon will consider many factors when deciding whether to remove both the tonsils and the adenoids or one or the other. However, if the patient is having both daytime and nighttime symptoms of sleep-disordered breathing, or has a sleep study showing obstructive sleep apnea, then removal of BOTH the tonsils and adenoids is generally recommended as first-line treatment.

What is drug-induced sleep endoscopy?

Drug-induced sleep endoscopy (abbreviated, DISE) is a scope evaluation performed with child asleep in the operating room. The DISE procedure allows the surgeon to look at different potential "sites of obstruction" that may be responsible for causing the obstructive sleep symptoms. During DISE, the child receives medication through an IV, which causes the child to enter into a sleep-like state. Once the child is asleep, a flexible scope is advanced from the front of the nose all the way down the back of the throat until the vocal cords are visible. The goal is not only to determine what sites may be causing the obstruction but also to decide if there is something that can be done to surgically correct it. The exam takes about 15 minutes, and the patient is asleep for the entire procedure. DISE is often used when patients continue to have obstructive sleep apnea even after their tonsils and adenoids have been removed, to check what other site or sites are causing the obstruction.

The potential "sites of obstruction" that can be assessed during DISE include:

- Inferior turbinate enlargement.
- Deviated septum.
- Enlarged adenoids.
- Soft palate/velum.
- Enlarged tonsils.
- Pharyngeal wall collapse.
- Lingual tonsils.
- Base of tongue collapse.
- Collapse of the cartilage structures above the vocal folds (laryngomalacia).

Below is a picture obtained during surgery of a child's enlarged turbinates.

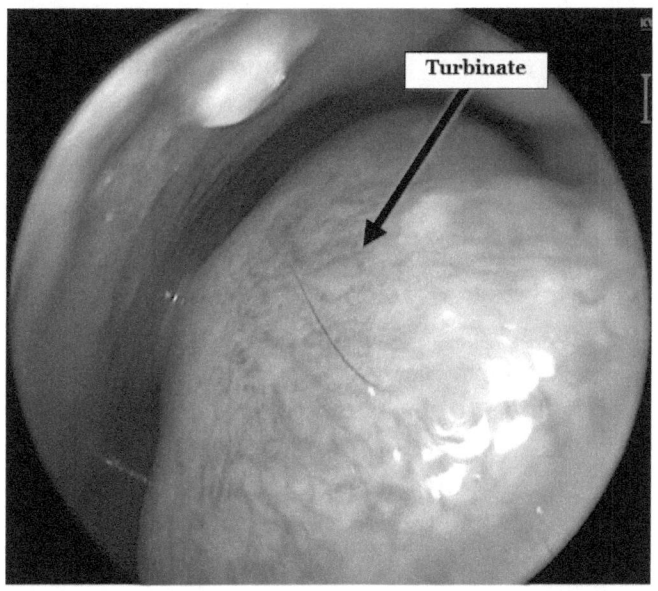

What are other surgeries for sleep apnea besides removal of tonsils and adenoids?

Although tonsils and adenoids are the most common structures to cause obstructive sleep apnea in children, there are several other "sites of obstruction" that can cause obstruction during sleep. As discussed above, DISE can often be helpful in determining which site(s) are contributing to the obstructive breathing. In some instances, surgery can be done to improve the obstructive site. The age of the child plays a role in determining which surgery the child may be a candidate for, as several of the surgeries listed below are only safe for older children.

- Inferior turbinate reduction is the process whereby the inferior turbinate in the nose is reduced in size to improve nasal airflow. Surgery is performed through the nostrils on both sides of the nose.
- Septoplasty is a surgery that corrects a displacement or deviation of the bone and cartilage that divides the two sides of the nose. This surgery is usually not recommended until the teenage years.
- Uvuloplasty is a surgery that can be done to modify and shorten the length of the uvula.
- Lingual tonsillectomy. Some children have tonsil tissue that grows on the very back of the tongue. This tonsil tissue is separate from the tonsils (palatine tonsils), which are in the back of the throat. A surgery can be done to remove this lingual tonsil tissue from the back of the tongue. The palatine and the lingual tonsils are removed at different times in order to prevent circumferential pharyngeal scarring.
- Base of tongue reduction is a procedure where a wedge of tissue from the very back of the tongue is removed to reduce the overall size of the base of the tongue. Having an enlarged base of tongue is a common site of obstruction, particularly in children with Down syndrome. This surgery is more commonly completed in older children with severe obstructive sleep

apnea.

- Supraglottoplasty is a surgery that is done through the mouth using scopes and cameras to address collapse of the cartilage structures above the vocal folds (laryngomalacia). This is the most common procedure completed for infants with obstructive breathing.

- Mandibular distraction osteogenesis is a surgery that lengthens a small jaw. This surgery is recommended mainly for infants with very small or short jaws who have obstructive sleep apnea.

- Uvulopalatopharyngoplasty (UPPP) is a surgery that removes or remodels tissue in the throat, mainly the uvula, soft palate, tonsils, and the pharynx. It is uncommonly performed in the pediatric age group.

- Tracheostomy is a surgical procedure that involves creating an opening through the neck to the windpipe or trachea to insert a breathing tube. This opening could be either permanent or temporary, depending on the underlying problem. This procedure is usually the last resort to treat obstructive sleep apnea.

OSA Surgery	Typical age when surgery is performed
Supraglottoplasty	0-12 months
Mandibular distraction osteogenesis	0-12 months
Adenoidectomy	12-24 months
Adenotonsillectomy	2-18 years
Uvuloplasty	4-18 years
Inferior turbinate reduction	1-18 years
Septoplasty	13-18 years
Uvuloplatopharyngoplasty	13-18 years
Lingual tonsillectomy	4-18 years
Base of tongue reduction	4-18 years
Tracheostomy	0 -18 years

References

1. Bitar MA, Dowli A, Mourad M. The effect of tonsillectomy on the immune system: A systematic review and meta-analysis. Int J Pediatr Otorhinolaryngol. 2015 Aug;79(8):1184-91.
2. Colclasure JB, Graham SS. Complications of outpatient tonsillectomy and adenoidectomy: a review of 3,340 cases. Ear Nose Throat J. 1990 Mar;69(3):155-60.
3. Duval M, Chung JC, Vaccani JP. A case-control study of repeated adenoidectomy in children. JAMA Otolaryngol Head Neck Surg. 2013 Jan;139(1):32-6.
4. Ingram DG, Ruiz AG, Gao D, Friedman NR. Success of Tonsillectomy for Obstructive Sleep Apnea in Children With Down Syndrome. J Clin Sleep Med. 2017 Aug 15;13(8):975-980.

6

CPAP FOR SLEEP APNEA
Tamika A. Cranford, RPSGT, RRT
Jane B. Taylor, MD

How does CPAP work?

Obstructive sleep apnea occurs due to repetitive partial or complete collapse of the upper airway during sleep. When this occurs, it is difficult to inhale oxygen and exhale carbon dioxide. The brain senses these changes, arouses your child from sleep, and the airway opens to resume normal breathing. CPAP (continuous positive airway pressure) is a machine that blows air into the airway. The extra air and pressure acts as a pneumatic (pressure) splint to prevent the upper airway from collapsing/closing. This helps maintain good airflow and normal breathing when you are sleeping.

How do I get a CPAP machine?

First, you see a sleep or pulmonary doctor who will ask lots of questions about your child's sleep and will do a physical exam. Based on the findings of this exam, the doctor will order a sleep study if your child is suspected to have sleep-disordered breathing. The sleep study is done overnight in a sleep lab. See Chapter 3 for further information on sleep studies. The sleep study monitors your child's breathing, oxygen and carbon dioxide levels, among several other things. If the sleep study shows your child has obstructive sleep apnea (OSA), then your physician will call you to talk about your options. If it is mild OSA, then it might be managed medically with nasal steroids and leukotriene inhibitors. If it is more severe, your doctor will discuss other management options. One option could include a referral to an ear, nose and throat (ENT) physician, who might recommend surgery. Another option is trialing a CPAP machine in the sleep lab during a second sleep study. Some patients require both surgical and CPAP interventions.

A mask fitting will be done to find the best fit for your child. Then, CPAP will be trialed in the sleep lab. When the correct pressure settings are established for your child, then the sleep physician will send an order for the CPAP machine to a durable medical equipment (DME) company. There are many different DME companies out in the community and your insurance company has contracts with some of them. You will be asked to call your insurance company to see what DME companies you can choose from. Once you have picked the best DME for you, then the physician will send the company the order. Upon approval from your insurance, the DME company will drop off the CPAP machine, tubing, mask, and supplies at your house and they should do teaching on the equipment with you. A repeat mask fitting can be done if your child did not find a comfortable mask option at the first mask fitting during the sleep study.

What are the different types of CPAP machines?

There are a surprising number of different modes on these machines.

CPAP (continuous positive airway pressure) delivers a constant flow of pressure during inhalation and exhalation. For example, a CPAP of 5cmH2o delivers an air pressure of 5cmH2o to the airway. In addition, the air pressure can be either a set number the entire night, or a range of numbers (auto-titrating CPAP, or APAP) that is used to keep your child's airway open so she sleeps well. When APAP is selected, the sleep provider will set the minimum and maximum pressures that the machine can deliver, and throughout the night the pressure may increase or decrease automatically based on if the machine senses pauses in breathing or not. For example, an APAP of 5-10cmH2O means that the machine will start at 5cmH2O of pressure, and can increase throughout the night to a maximum of 10cmH2O. APAP is much more often used in adults than in children. Figuring out if this mode works as well or better compared to regular CPAP is an active area of research.

BPAP (bi-level positive airway pressure) delivers a higher pressure during inhalation and a lower pressure during exhalation. Therefore, there are two different numbers to set. For example, a BPAP of 12/8cmH2O means that the machine delivers 12cmH2O during inhalation and 8cmH2O during exhalation. BPAP is a mode that is more often used if a child has difficulty taking deep breaths during sleep, for example, if he has muscle weakness due to muscular dystrophy. It is also sometimes used if a patient has problems adjusting to CPAP or needs high pressures.

There are other modes of BPAP that are also used to help treat more complex sleep apneas. These include:

BPAP ST (spontaneous/timed) is exactly the same as BPAP discussed above, except that a backup rate is added, meaning that if the machine detects a pause in breathing, it will deliver the pressure, effectively giving the patient a breath. This mode can assist children with breathing by making sure they are taking an adequate number of breaths per minute, and is therefore sometimes used to treat central sleep apnea.

BPAP ASV (adaptive servo ventilation) mode also delivers a higher pressure during inhalation and a lower pressure during exhalation, similar to the other modes of BPAP. It also has a backup rate. What is different is that the machine will analyze your child's pattern of breathing, and will automatically adjust either or both the lower (exhalation) and higher (inhalation) pressures throughout the night to stabilize the respiratory pattern. This mode is most often used for central sleep apnea, periodic breathing, and complex (both obstructive and central components) sleep apnea.

BPAP AVAPS (average volume assured pressure support) mode is fundamentally different than the other modes discussed above in that it focuses on the volume of air delivered (hence "volume assured") rather than the pressure of air delivered. This mode can be helpful for children who have difficulty taking sufficiently deep breaths during sleep, such as children with muscular dystrophy. BPAP AVAPS is unique in that it can adjust the inspiratory pressure given to the child based on measured volumes of air that are exhaled, ensuring that adequate amounts of air are given over time.

What are the machine features?

There are a few different features on your machine depending on the manufacturer. They all have an on/off button, a LED screen, and turn knob to allow you to access your settings. This is where you will find the humidity control and be able to see what setting you are on. You will also be able to check the mask fit on this screen to make sure it is fitting properly and not leaking. Some have a triangle button on top (ramp button), that if pushed, lowers the pressure to make it more comfortable for your child to start wearing the CPAP. Other machines will automatically ramp without pushing the button. Some have different alarms that may be set, and they all have Wi-Fi and Bluetooth capabilities that allow you to track how your child is doing with the machine on your smartphone with an app or on your computer.

On the following pages, a typical CPAP device is shown to demonstrate the typical features and settings. Your particular machine may be a different model or brand, so consult your owner's manual for your particular machine. Please note that as the patient you can change certain settings on your machine (such as humidification), but some settings can only be changed by your physician. The white boxes have been added to conceal the brand name of the machine.

The picture below is a typical CPAP machine. Note that the user is turning the machine on by pressing the power button.

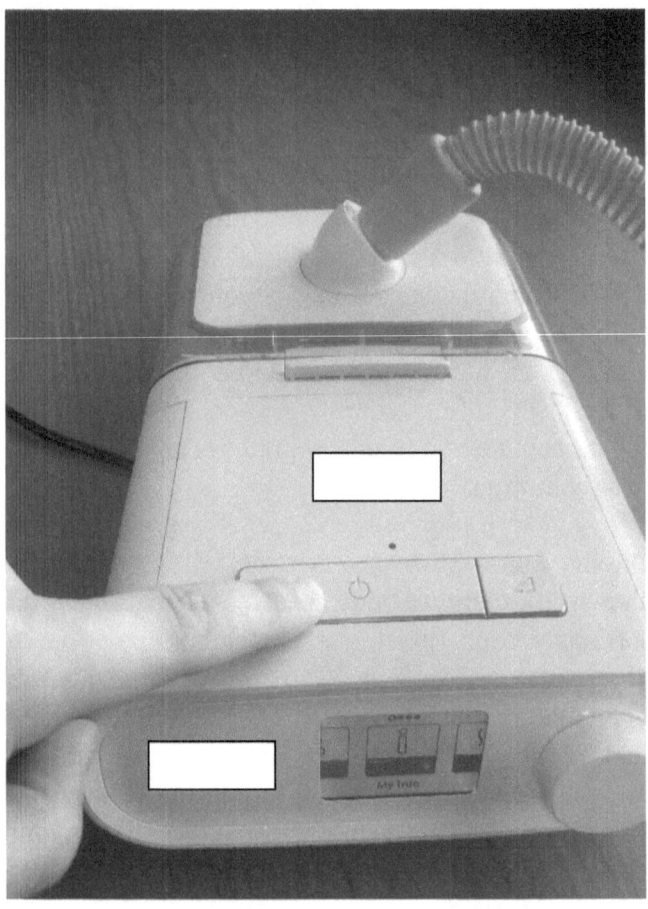

Don't forget to fill the humidification chamber with distilled water!

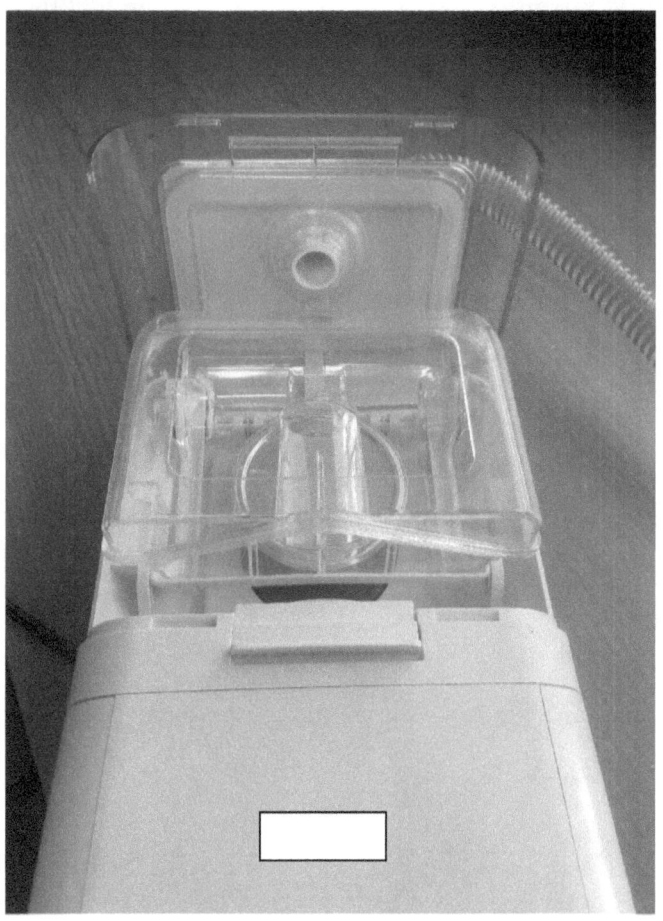

Press the triangle-shaped button to start the "ramp" feature, which will start the CPAP at a lower pressure and gradually ramp up to the therapeutic pressure. This can sometimes make it easier to fall asleep with the CPAP on.

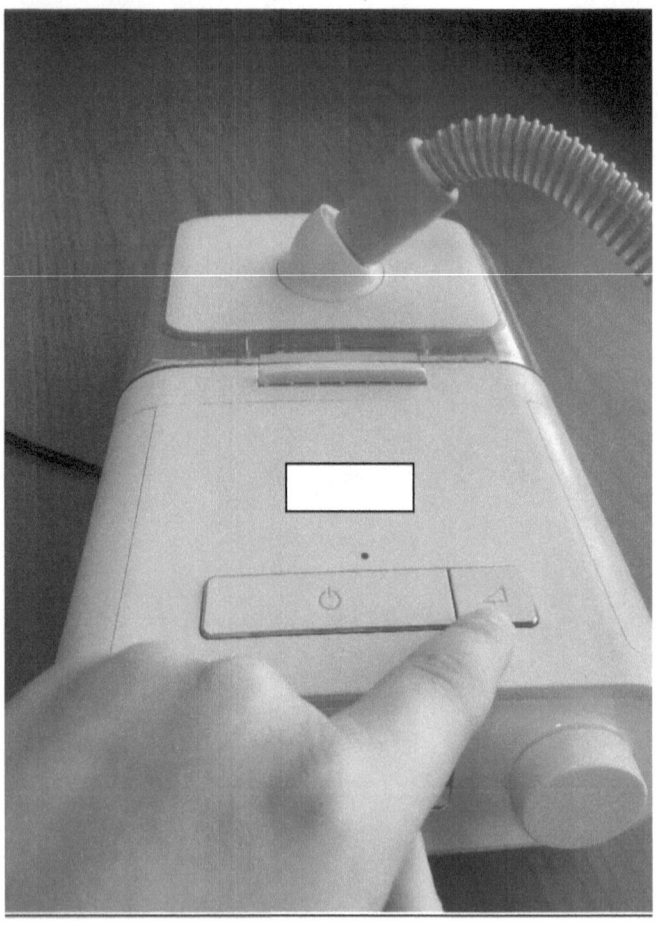

Note that the CPAP machine needs to be plugged into a power source to work.

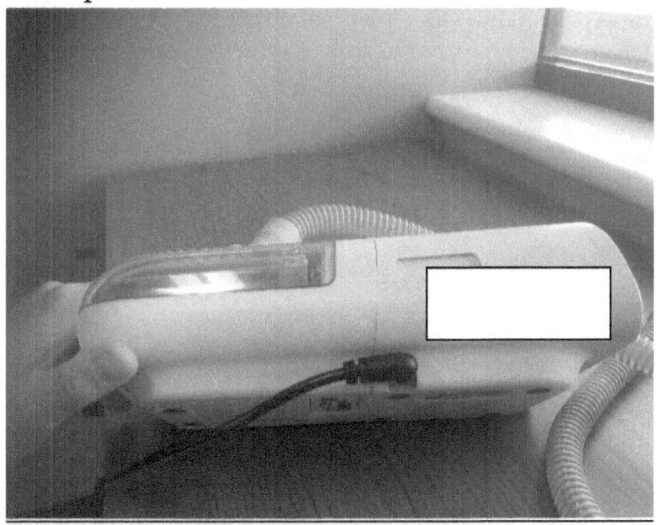

From the "My Info" screen you can view a lot of information.

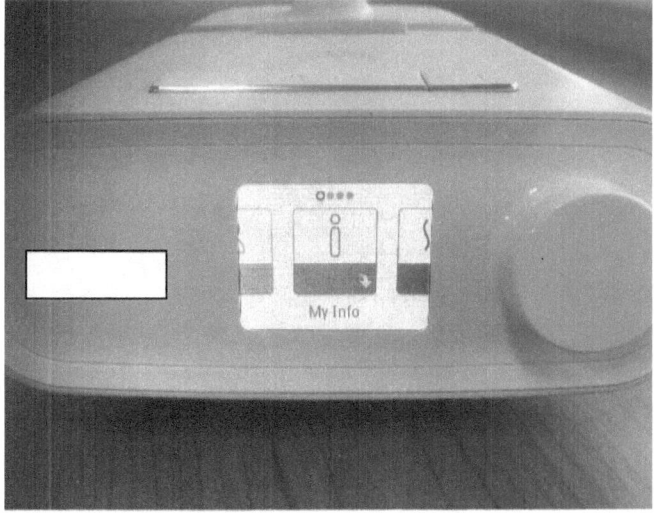

The therapy hours tells you how often your child has been using the CPAP.

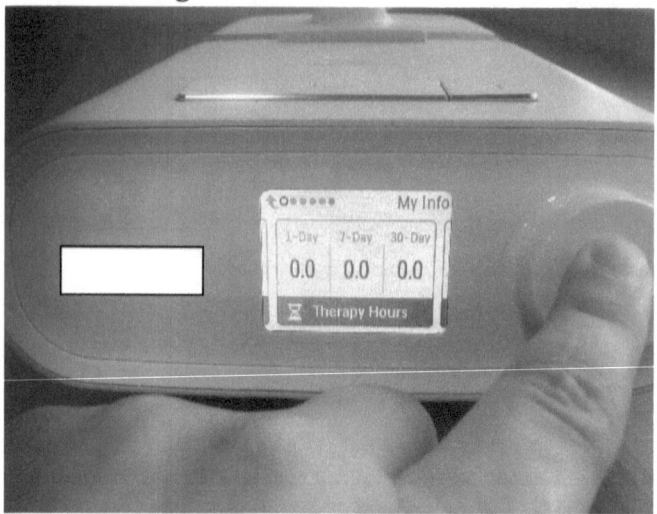

The AHI gives you an estimate of how well the machine is controlling your child's sleep apnea.

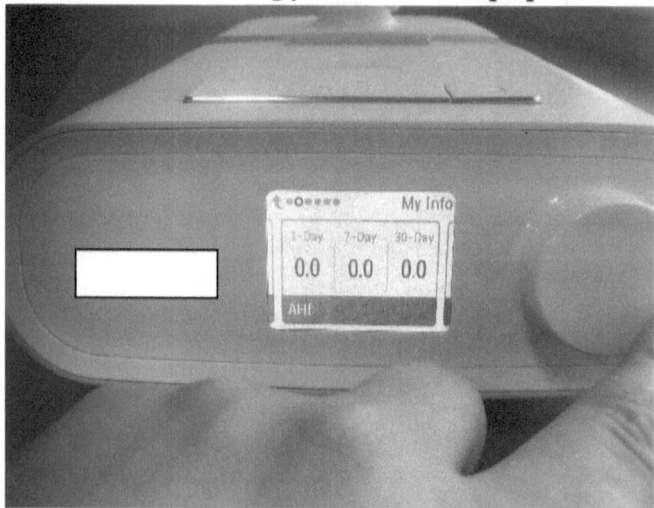

The mask fit screen lets you know if the machine detects large leak around the mask.

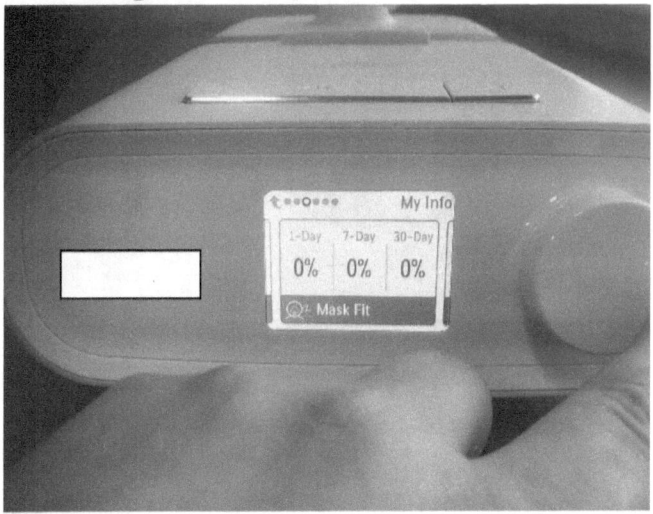

The machine records if your child is having periodic breathing (irregular breathing with apneas).

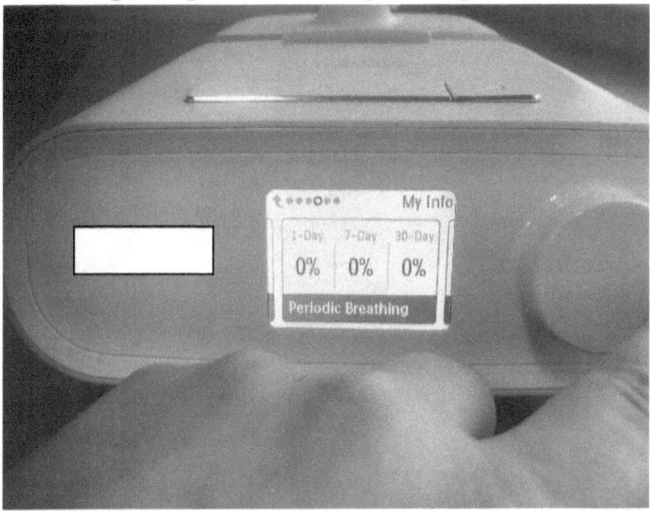

If your child is using APAP, the 90% pressure tells you that the machine was giving that pressure or lower 90% of the night.

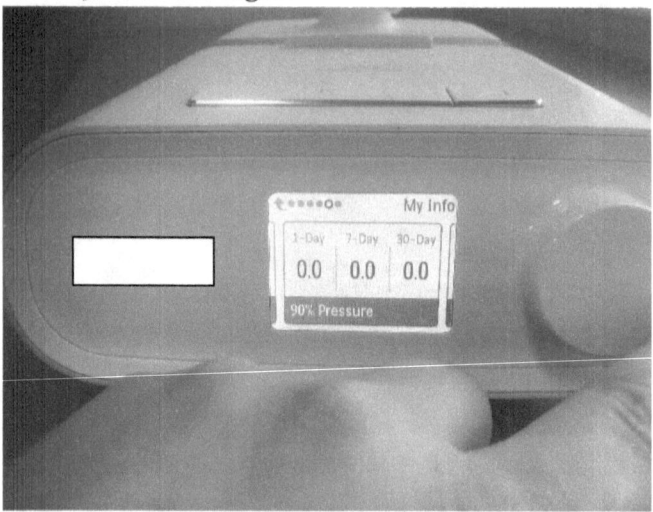

The preheat feature can heat the water tank of the humidifier in advance to increase comfort.

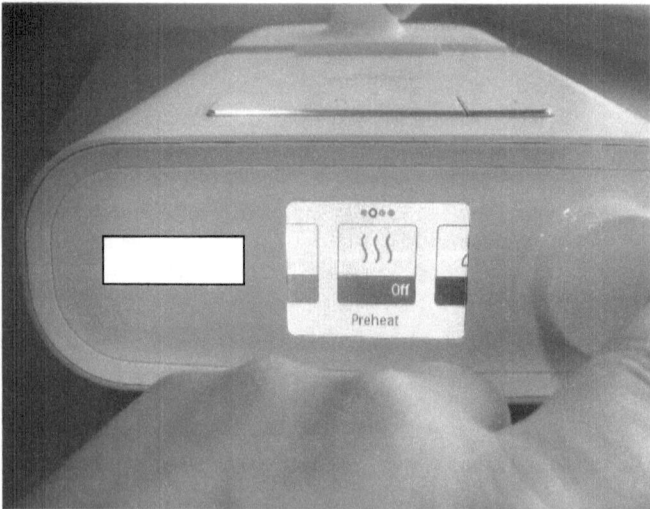

The "My Provider" menu allows you to see information regarding your device and provider contact information.

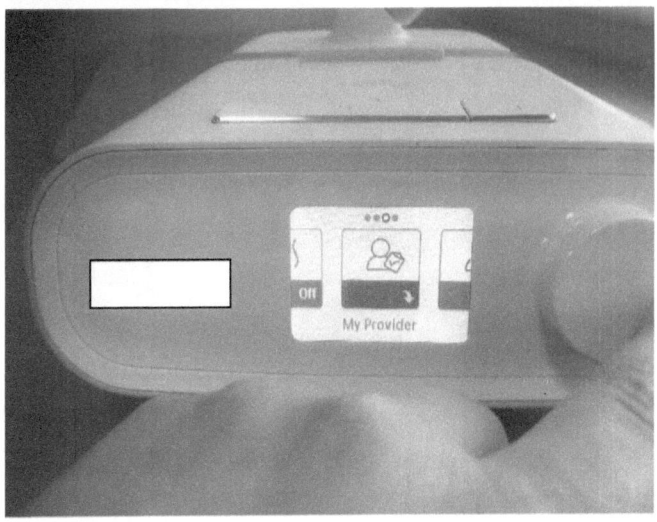

Under "My Setup," you can change several settings.

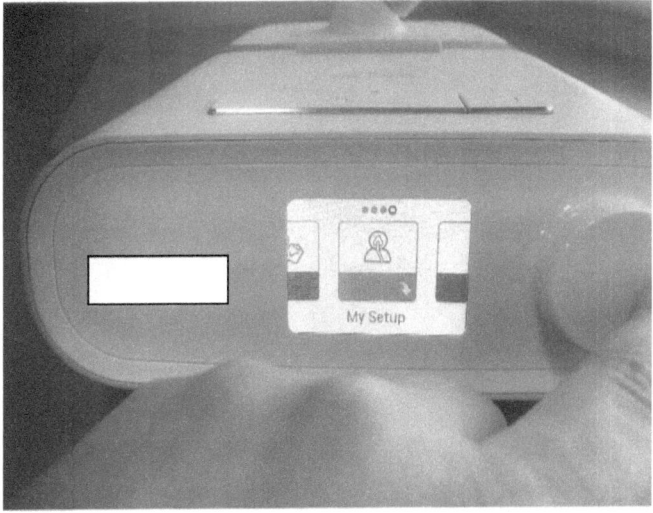

You can set the ramp starting pressure and ramp time.

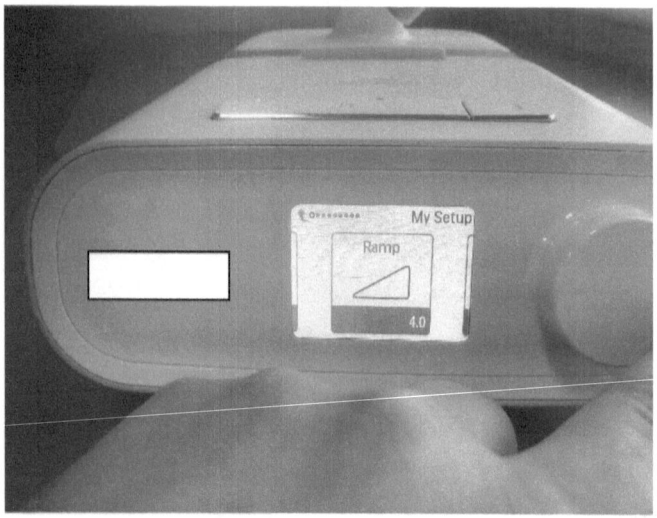

FLEX allows you to adjust the pressure relief (less pressure during exhalation for comfort).

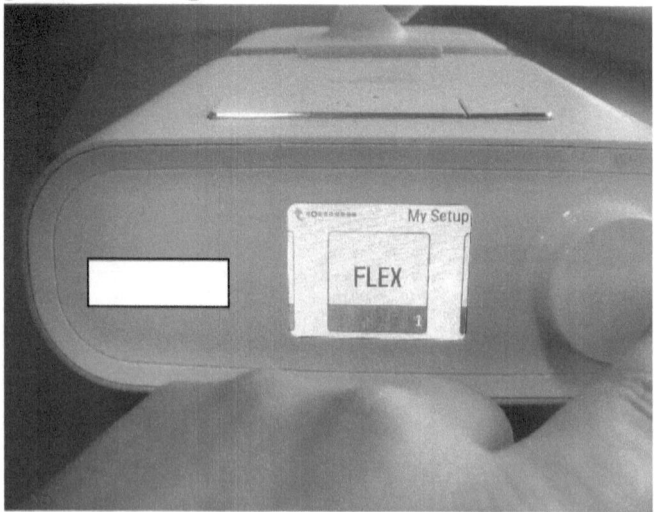

The heater can adapt to the room temperature to minimize condensation.

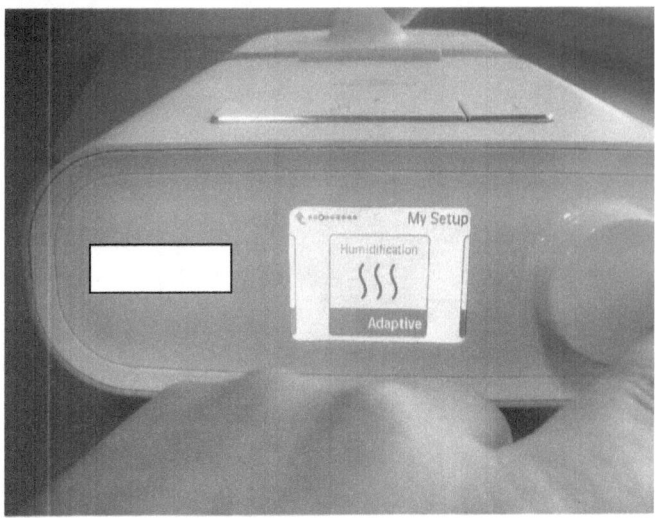

Selecting your mask type allows the machine to adjust the level of pressure relief.

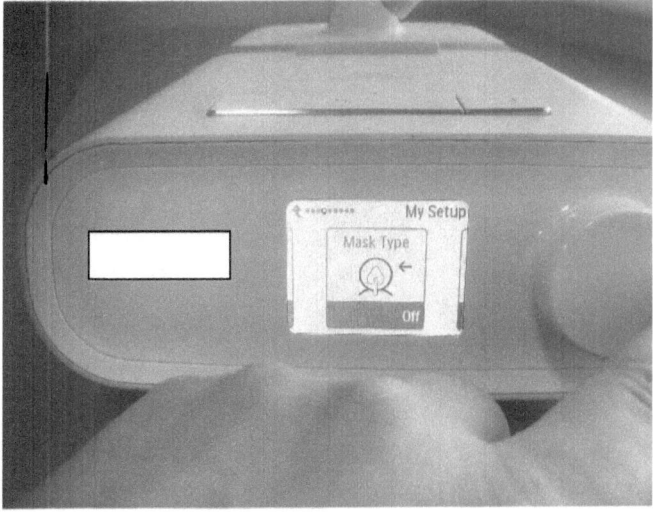

You select the diameter size of the tubing you are using and if it is heated tubing.

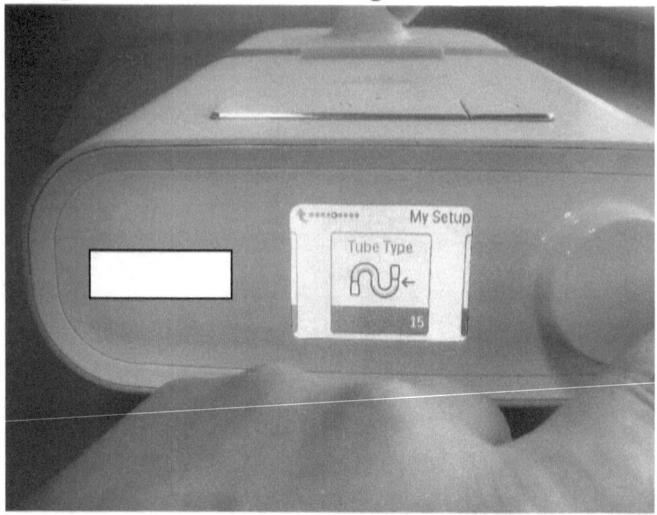

You can choose your preferred language.

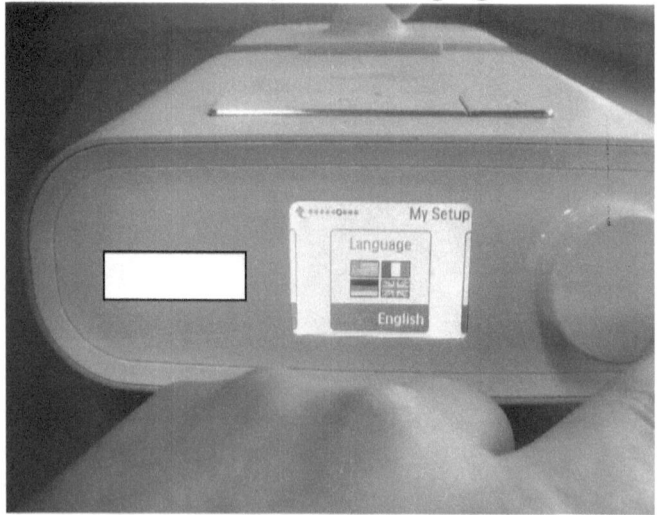

You can turn the machine modem on or off.

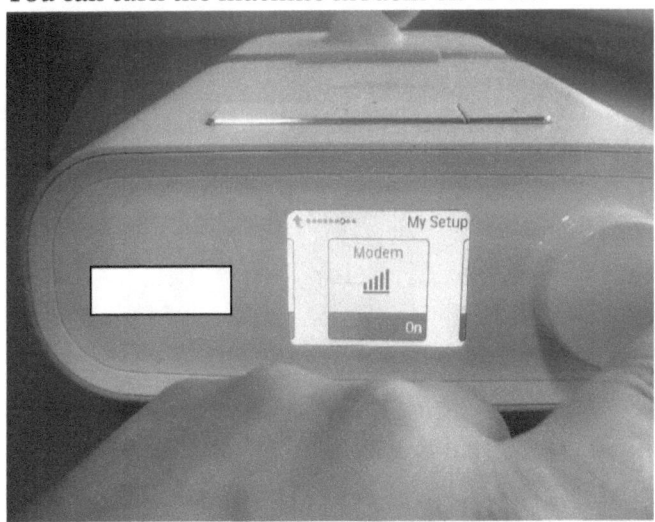

You can turn the Bluetooth feature on or off. Most machines can now be paired to your mobile device and you can review your data with an app.

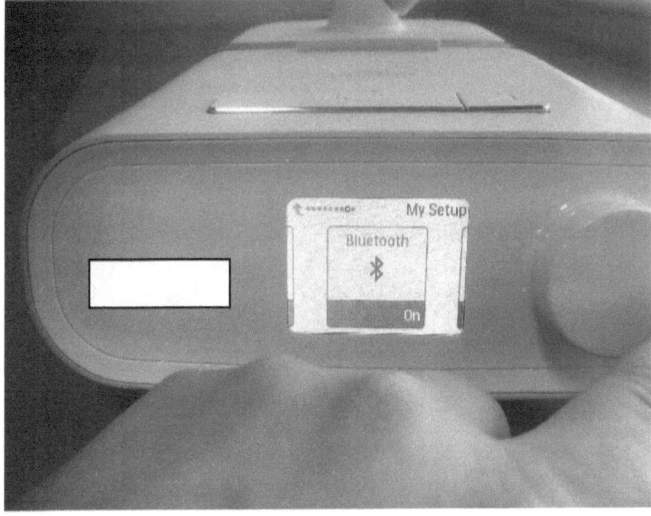

You can adjust the time.

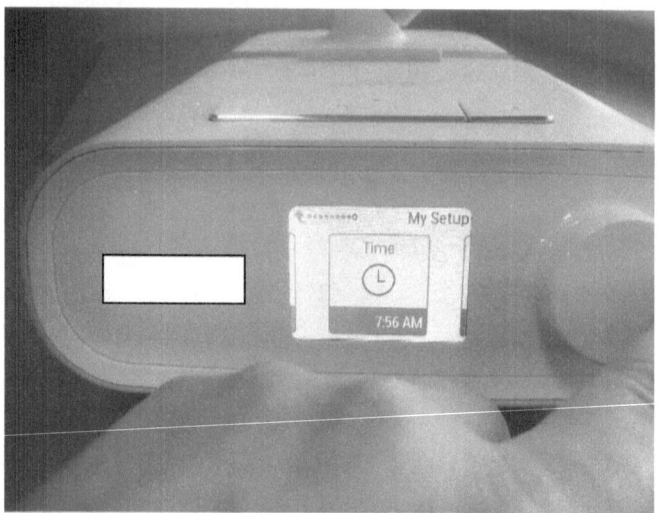

The air filter will need to be replaced periodically.

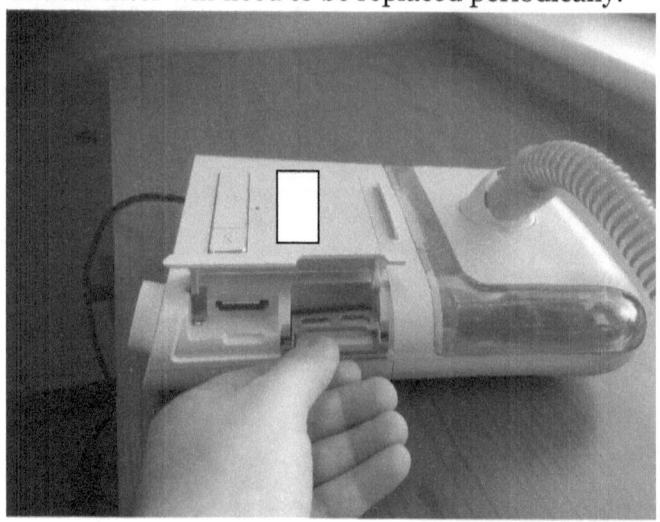

The SD card contains all of the data from your machine. Your provider may download that data during your visit, so be sure to bring this card (or your entire machine) to your CPAP follow-up visits.

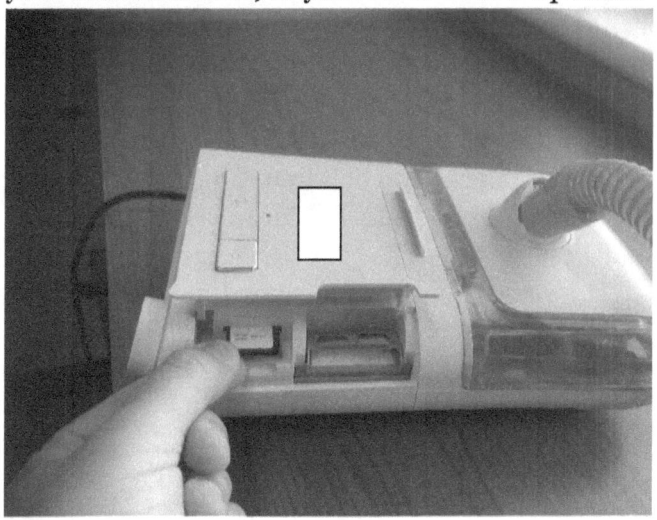

How do I take care of my CPAP?

Follow the manufacturer's guidelines for cleaning. The mask and headgear should be cleaned daily. The tubing and humidifier should be cleaned once a week. Filters need to be changed at least once a month. Clean your equipment with a basic dish soap like Dawn or Palmolive, without any antibacterial substance (because it will break down the mask quicker). If your child has sensitive skin, a detergent like Dreft without dyes or perfumes is recommended. Hang your tubing over the shower rod to make sure all the water drains out. Use only distilled water in your humidifier. The humidifier should be emptied any time you travel with your CPAP (or BPAP) so the machine doesn't get water damage.

What are the different mask types and which one is right for my child?

Many different types of CPAP masks are available for use in infants and children. The masks fall into three major categories: full face mask, nasal mask, and nasal pillows. The full face mask covers both the nose and mouth at the same time. Some of the full face masks cover the eyes too and look like a scuba mask. Other full face masks only cover the nose and mouth like the mask a fighter pilot wears. All full face masks run a risk of aspiration if the child vomits into the mask. Aspiration is where food or secretions are accidentally breathed into the airway. Aspiration can cause pneumonia and damage to the lungs. For this reason, a nasal mask or nasal pillows are tried first for most children. However, some children cannot close their mouths and so cannot be properly ventilated with the CPAP when the pressure escapes through their mouth. In these cases, the full face mask is used.

The nasal mask covers just the nose of the child. This mask is the most commonly used mask for children and is normally well tolerated. As the child grows and his nostrils increase in size, then nasal pillow masks can be considered. The nasal pillow masks do not completely surround the nose;

instead, they seal off the opening to the nose (nostrils) and are much smaller and tend to involve less tubing than the traditional nasal mask. Many teenagers prefer the nasal pillows once their nose is large enough for this mask type.

If ever you feel your child's mask is not fitting properly or your child is old enough to tell you they do not like their mask, another mask fitting may be performed by a sleep clinic specialist if there is one at your location or by the DME provider. It is recommended that you go to the DME provider for the fitting as you will have more mask choices.

There are a variety of different mask types to choose from. Below are examples of some common mask types, including a nasal masks (top panels), full facemasks (bottom left), and total facemask (bottom right).

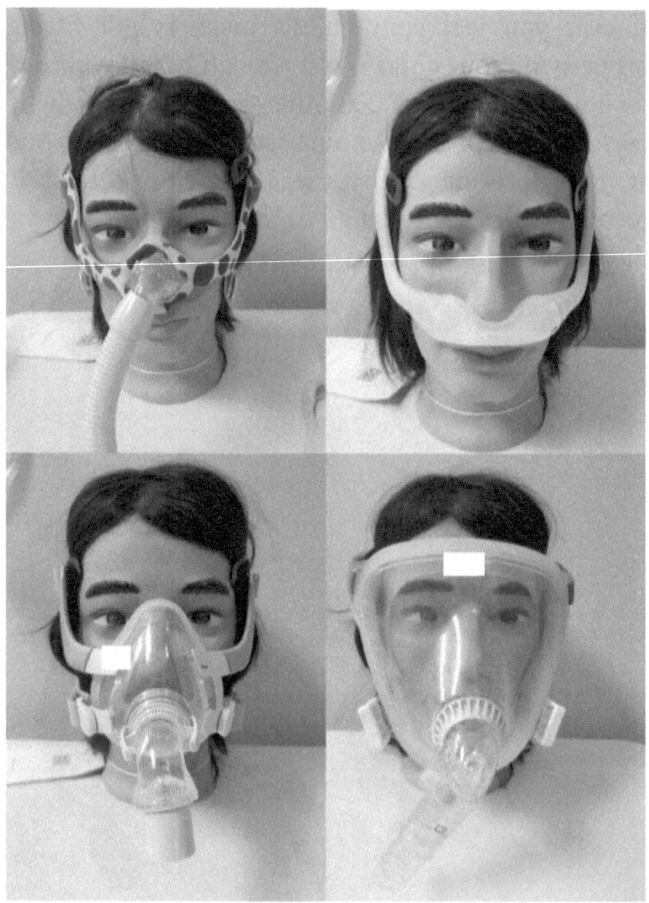

How do I deal with...?

Too much pressure: Sometimes a child's CPAP needs change over time. If you suspect that there is too much pressure, then calling your sleep or pulmonary provider is the first step. One issue that can appear like there is too much pressure is actually an ill-fitting mask. An ill-fitting mask causes air to leak, which can be uncomfortable and lead to dry eyes. Your sleep or pulmonary physician will likely call the DME company to send a respiratory therapist (RT) out to your home. The RT will check the mask's fit and settings of your CPAP machine. If the mask is fitting well and the machine is working properly, then another sleep study may be ordered to re-titrate the machine and find the pressure settings that work for your child at that time. Remember, as your child grows and her medical condition changes, the CPAP settings will also change.

Dry Mouth: Some children develop dry mouth while on CPAP. There is a humidity setting that allows the CPAP machine to deliver warm, humidified air to your child. This helps combat the dry mouth/nasal passages and can be adjusted as needed. Sometimes, if the humidity is increased to help with dryness, the warm air can condense into water in the tubing between the machine and mask; this is called "rainout." Because the basic cause of rainout is that the heated humidified air in the tube is warmer than the air in the room, you can decrease rainout by decreasing humidity or temperature level of your machine (but this may result in dryness again), by increasing room temperature (but this may affect your child's ability to fall asleep), by using a tube cover or wrap to insulate the tubing and keep the heat in, or by obtaining a heated tube (contains a heated coil) from your DME company. If your child continues to have issues with dry mouth or if water continues to build up in the CPAP circuit, then alerting your DME company and sleep or pulmonary provider is important so the machine can be adjusted.

Mask Leak: As your child grows, her face changes in shape and size. For this reason, the mask that worked well last year may not be the best mask this year. If the mask begins to leak, then your provider will order another mask fitting to see what change needs to occur in the mask. You may be given a different type of mask or the same mask but in a larger size. It is important to have a properly fitting mask. An improperly fitted mask could affect the pressure that needs to be delivered to your child's airway to help maintain good air movement in the lungs when she is asleep. If the mask leaks, then not all of the pressure is going to the airway to help support it.

Skin Irritation: Masks can be irritating to the skin. The skin irritation can be from rubbing, moisture, or development of a skin allergy to the plastic in the mask. To help with skin irritation from a mask that is putting pressure on certain facial structures or rubbing, two things can be done. Mepilex, a soft adhesive fabric, can be prescribed and cut into the shape of the area of skin that is irritated. The Mepilex provides a barrier between the mask and skin and offers extra padding to protect the face. There are also commercial barriers that can be obtained online that are fit specifically for your mask (called CPAP mask liners). Your provider may also order a second type of mask that fits differently and can be alternated with the first mask to cut down on skin irritation produced by the first mask when used on a nightly basis. Skin irritation by moisture can sometimes occur from applying moisturizers to the skin right before the CPAP mask is placed. For this reason, it is not recommended to use skin moisturizers right before bed; instead, use them in the morning. If the humidity in the CPAP machine is too high, it can also cause some moisture around the mask seal on the face. If this is the case, the humidification settings on your CPAP machine can be turned down. Finally, some individuals develop a skin allergy to the plastic in the masks. If a skin allergy develops, then a cloth mask can be prescribed for the CPAP machine. There are many different mask options out there, so it is extremely rare not be able to find one that works well for your child over time. Be patient and don't get frustrated if your child needs to try out a few different masks before finding one that works the best for her; and, remember, over time the mask will need to be changed as the child grows.

How do I travel with CPAP?

Your machine will come with a travel bag. Several accessories specific to your equipment can be purchased so you can use your machine while traveling. There are car chargers, battery packs, and converters. They vary in price depending on which ones you want. Make sure you read the descriptions thoroughly, especially for battery packs. They come in different sizes and can only meet certain pressures. With most batteries, you will not be able to use your humidifier. Everything will fit nicely in your travel bag. Make sure you empty your water chamber before you travel with it. If you decide to purchase any accessories for travel, make sure they are compatible with your machine. Your DME company will be to help you by looking up your model number if needed.

If you are flying with your CPAP, we recommend taking it as a carry-on item, so it has less chance of being damaged. You will likely need to remove the CPAP from its case when you go through security, and you may want to consider bringing your child's CPAP prescription or letter of medical necessity with you. Because your CPAP machine is necessary medical equipment, it should not be counted towards your carry-on limits.

How do I work well with my DME provider?

Working well with your DME provider starts with

the first call you make to them. You will want to verify they take your insurance, take pediatric patients (some do not and some only take patients above a certain weight), and can answer other questions you may have. You may want to ask them how often you can get replacement supplies. The company should be able to give you a list of how often you can get different supplies. You should also find out if you have to contact the company to order supplies or if they contact you, or if automatic shipping can be set up. If you are having problems with your equipment, contact the company immediately so they can help address the issues. It can be helpful to write down notes during phone conversations so that you remember what you were told and can reference them in the future. Remember that the DME companies are many times handling high volumes of patients, so do your best to remain patient while still advocating for your child. In addition, some sleep clinics have a specialist (CPAP coordinator or educator) that can also help with issues you may be having, whether with the mask, with using the CPAP, or with the DME company. If you are unhappy with your DME company, you can always switch to another one, but unless you get a new machine, the new company will not make adjustments to your equipment.

What if my child cannot tolerate CPAP?

There are many reasons why people do not tolerate CPAP. Sometimes it is as simple as changing the mask, while other times it is a matter of getting the child used to the new machine and bedtime routine. Talk with your provider or specialist about things that can be done to help with desensitization, a gradual process of getting your child used to wearing the mask and having positive airflow present when she is asleep (see Chapter 7 for a detailed discussion). Your provider or specialist can also order a mask fitting so you and your child can trial different masks to get one that fits well and is comfortable. Features on the machines can be adjusted to help make it more tolerable to wear; for example, the ramp feature allows for the pressure to start low and slowly increase over several minutes so it is not as intense right when the mask is put on. There are also psychologists specializing in sleep medicine who are trained to help with the lifestyle changes and desensitization issues if they cannot be easily managed by you and your sleep provider alone. Non-invasive ventilation is a big change in lifestyle for a child, but if introduced in a supportive manner over time, it is usually tolerated. However, there are instances when parents and care providers do everything right and still the child cannot tolerate the non-invasive ventilator support (CPAP). In these rare cases, other options can be tried to address a child's sleep problems. There are dental and oral devices that can be worn. There are even some facial and throat exercises (myofunctional therapy) that have been shown to help with sleep-disordered breathing in specific individuals. If there are still sites of obstruction in the airway after surgery to remove the tonsils and adenoids, then the ENT or plastic surgeon may decide to perform another surgery like tongue reduction, mandibular distraction, or tracheostomy placement.

7

HELPING CHILDREN WEAR CPAP
Kevin C. Smith, PhD, CBSM

Now that you have information about sleep apnea and the importance of CPAP treatment, you are probably wondering how you are going to get your child to wear CPAP. You are not alone! In the beginning, using CPAP can be challenging. Here are a few tips:

Anticipate some initial frustration. It is normal for children to need time to adjust to having a chronic illness that requires daily treatment. During this period, your child may feel fear, anger, embarrassment, confusion, or resentment about having sleep apnea and needing CPAP therapy. Although this should not prevent you and your child from moving forward with treatment, your support and empathy will make it easier.

Make CPAP a consistent part of the bedtime routine. Putting on the CPAP mask should either be the last step of the bedtime routine, or come right before an in-bed activity that involves your presence, such as reading a story.

You may need to **sit next to your child's bed** for the first several nights he wears CPAP. This is especially true if your child takes off the mask when you leave. Other children need extra support until they get used to CPAP therapy, but stay only if they ask you to, and avoid getting into your child's bed if possible. Now this may seem like a step backwards if you usually leave the room before your child is asleep. Just explain to your child that this is a temporary change. Additionally, your child may only need "check-ins," where you leave the room for a few minutes and return briefly to see how he is doing.

Your child can be successful at wearing CPAP without being perfect. Of course, wearing CPAP every night, all night is optimal, and more usage means better treatment outcomes. But everyone has an occasional "off night" (see CPAP challenges below). You and your child's medical team can discuss realistic CPAP usage goals so you can provide your child with clear expectations. And if your child's therapy is going really well, you and your child's doctors may decide an occasional

"CPAP holiday" is appropriate for a special occasion, such as a sleepover at a friend's house. That said, your child may feel so good after wearing CPAP that she won't want to miss a night.

Plan ahead for known schedule changes. If you are a two-household family with one CPAP machine, it will take coordination and planning for consistent use between homes. Vacations or overnight visits with relatives also take extra preparation.

Avoid using CPAP therapy as a punishment or reward. Examples: "Since you did not do your homework, you will have to wear CPAP every night this week." Or, "Since you ate your vegetables, you do not have to wear CPAP tonight." (This is different than an occasional break, like for a one-night sleepover, mentioned above.)

Use the support of extended family members. What child does not like a social media message, text, phone call or visit from an aunt, grandparent, or other relative telling her she is doing a great job wearing her CPAP?

Use a CPAP buddy. Ask your CPAP team if they have a "buddy" program to connect your child with other CPAP users to get firsthand advice and support. A friend or family member that consistently uses CPAP can also be a great resource.

Celebrate CPAP victories. Have you noticed that your child is less tired during the day or that behaviors have improved since wearing CPAP? Let her know! She may be feeling better as well, but might not associate this improvement with using CPAP. This may be very important to teens, because improved functioning during the day could result in added benefits, such as better grades or the ability to get a driver's license.

BUT MY CHILD STILL WON'T WEAR IT.

Even with a comprehensive CPAP therapy plan in place, CPAP usage is still challenging for many children and their families. So if you are finding that you are struggling, you are not alone. Below are some suggestions to address some of the more common challenges:

The mask is still uncomfortable even after the initial mask fitting.

One of the most common reasons for not wearing CPAP is an uncomfortable mask. Often it is difficult to really know how a mask is going to feel or perform until you actually use it at home for a few nights. Keep an eye out for any air leaks, skin abrasions on the face as a result of the mask rubbing, or other concerns. Do not be afraid to reach out to your home health care company or prescribing physician to get help with these problems. Your child is much more likely to use

CPAP if the mask fits properly.

Your child is afraid of the mask or thinks he won't be able to breathe with it on.

Some kids are just afraid of CPAP – the machine, the mask, everything about it. If this is your child, exposure therapy (sometimes known as "desensitization") may be helpful. The goal of exposure therapy is to gradually expose a child to the feared object (in this case, the CPAP machine or mask) without any danger, in order to overcome anxiety and/or distress. Below is a sample exposure program plus additional recommendations to address CPAP usage. You can start with any step based on your child's current needs and level of comfort. Also, providing a distraction during the process during the first few steps, such as letting your child watch his favorite video, can be helpful. Finally, you may want to try the first few steps during the day, when your child likely will be more relaxed and rested.

Step 1. Let your child touch the mask and the unplugged machine. Depending on your child's age, you may want to decorate the CPAP machine and mask to make them less intimidating. You can find many creative ideas on the internet, but here's a quick and easy project: make the mask look like the head of an elephant by gluing two eyes and ears on it. (The hose already looks like an elephant's trunk.)

Step 2. Next, help or encourage your child to hold the CPAP mask on his face (disconnected completely from the machine) for brief amounts of time (maybe 5-10 seconds at first), then take a break. You could also take turns holding it on your face as well. Provide frequent encouragement and remind your child to breathe normally. As comfort levels increase, attach the mask straps and place the mask on your child's face (still unattached from the machine). Practice a few times a day, continuing to increase time intervals until your child can comfortably wear the mask for 20-30 minutes.

Step 3. Then, turn the machine on to its lowest setting and let your child feel the air flow coming into the mask with his hand. Help or encourage your child to hold the mask to his face. Once comfortable, turn the machine off and attach the mask to your child's face, then turn it back on. Have your child practice a few times a day wearing the mask, continuing to increase time intervals until your child can comfortably wear the mask for 20-30 minutes.

Step 4. Now you are ready for the bedroom. With your child in the bed, place the mask on her face and turn on the machine. Remind her to relax and breathe normally. In the beginning, you may need to sit next to the bed until your child falls asleep to ensure that the mask remains on.

Step 5. If your child is consistently falling asleep

with the CPAP mask on at bedtime but takes it off before morning, you may need to check periodically during the night – at least for the first few weeks. If so, keep in mind that some parents struggle to hear the air pressure if the mask is off. One strategy is to put a baby monitor next to the CPAP machine. Or you may want to set your alarm 3–4 hours after your child falls asleep to check.

Step 6. If your child takes the mask off in the middle of the night: first shut the machine off, then attempt put the mask back on your child without waking him. Then turn the machine back on. If your child wakes, briefly explain that her mask came off and that you are putting it back on. For the first few weeks, you may need to sit next to the bed until your child falls back to sleep to ensure it stays on.

Your child is not afraid of the mask, she just doesn't want to wear it.

Initially, few children are excited about CPAP therapy, but some children are more resistant than others. Every caregiver has a list of non-negotiable rules (like having to wear a seatbelt). You may find that moving CPAP therapy into this category in your mind can help you to utilize the behavioral strategies you use in other non-negotiable situations. Set firm and consistent CPAP usage goals. If your toddler pulls the mask off his face, replace it. For children over age 4 years, you may want to consider using a reward program to increase adherence. Rewards do not need to be big (or expensive) to be effective. In fact, for young children, small but frequent prizes (say, every other day), may be more effective than a larger prize they wait weeks to receive. Older children can more easily delay gratification and may only need a reward every several days to increase adherence. Privileges count as prizes too, and are more economical. You can use something as simple as a sticker chart to measure progress. There are many books and resources on the internet available to help you set up a reward program if you have never used one. With preteen and teens, focusing on the benefits of CPAP usage may help to increase motivation and improve CPAP usage.

Your child forgets to put it on.

Children frequently forget to put on CPAP (more so with teens). This problem is usually the result of using the bed for an activity other than sleep (like reading, watching television, doing homework) and falling asleep before putting on the mask. A straightforward solution: Use the bed only for sleep, and make sure the mask is on before getting into bed. This strategy could require a significant adjustment for some children who use their bed for other activities, so they will need your help finding alternate places in your home to study and relax.

8

SPECIAL KIDS
Zarmina Ehsan, MD
Jane B. Taylor, MD

Down syndrome

Children with Down syndrome (or Trisomy 21) are at increased risk for obstructive sleep apnea (OSA), with about 50%-100% having OSA. The high prevalence is likely because the bodies of children with Down syndrome can have several differences that predispose to sleep apnea, including a different facial structure, large tongue, low muscle tone, and obesity.

We know from research that history reported by parents is not sufficient for ruling out sleep apnea in these children. This basically means that the absence of the report of snoring does not mean absence of underlying obstructive sleep apnea. A recent study illustrating this point in children with Down syndrome compared those children with snoring, apneas, or restless sleep at least 6 nights per week with those children who had symptoms less than 3 nights per week; the frequency of symptoms did not predict the presence or absence or sleep apnea nor sleep apnea severity when present[1]. As a result, the American Academy of Pediatrics recommends that all children with Down syndrome have a sleep study by their fourth birthday regardless of symptoms. Your general pediatrician may refer you to a sleep clinic to get this done.

The options for treatment of sleep apnea are the same as in children without Down syndrome, with adenotonsillectomy the most common first step (refer to Chapter 4). The major difference in children with Down syndrome is that a large proportion of them do not achieve complete cure with adenotonsillectomy alone (up to 50% still have moderate or severe disease after surgery)[2]. The lower surgical cure rate is likely because there are typically several factors contributing to their airway obstruction beyond the tonsils and adenoids. Children with Down syndrome have a large tongue and have weaker muscle tone in general, which includes their neck and airway muscles. Even if the sleep apnea is not completely cured with removal of the tonsils and adenoids, most children do achieve improvement in their disease severity (for example, going from severe sleep apnea to moderate or mild sleep apnea). Other surgical options for children with Down syndrome who have had their tonsils and adenoids removed include tongue surgery, surgery on the palate, nose surgery, and facial advancement procedures (see Chapter 5); drug-induced sleep endoscopy is typically used to determine which, if any, of these procedures would be helpful for a particular child.

Prader-Willi syndrome

Children with Prader-Willi syndrome are at increased risk of obstructive sleep apnea due to their distinct craniofacial anatomy, low muscle tone, and obesity, with approximately 80% having OSA[3]. It is important to assess for obstructive sleep apnea especially if they have symptoms of snoring, breathing difficulty at night, or difficulty staying asleep. Because of their obesity and craniofacial anatomy, these children are also more likely to still have sleep apnea even after removal of the tonsils and adenoids. These children may also have central sleep apnea due to neurologic differences as well as altered responses to changes in CO_2 and oxygen levels.

Growth hormone is often prescribed to these children by the endocrinologist. There may be an increased risk of death in Prader-Willi syndrome patients who are taking growth hormone and have undiagnosed and untreated severe obstructive sleep apnea. Therefore, your endocrinologist will likely want to assess for sleep apnea prior to starting growth hormone. If sleep apnea is diagnosed, your endocrinologist will likely want it adequately treated prior to starting growth hormone therapy.

In addition to sleep apnea, children with Prader-Willi syndrome have an increased prevalence of narcolepsy (up to 35%)[3]. This increased prevalence may be due to hypothalamic abnormalities associated with the syndrome, although this is not well understood. Your sleep doctor can test for narcolepsy and, if diagnosed, prescribe medications that can improve daytime alertness.

Achondroplasia

Children with achondroplasia have several potential differences that can increase their risk for breathing abnormalities during sleep, with up to 75% having some form of sleep-disordered breathing[4]. First, children with achondroplasia may have a narrowing at the base of their skull that can result in compression of the brain stem, called foramen magnum stenosis. If the brain stem is compressed, this can affect a part of the brain called the medulla that helps control the drive to breathe, resulting in central apneas. In addition, compression of the brain stem can also affect the nerves that control muscles of the upper airway, and therefore result in obstructive apneas. Second, children with achondroplasia tend to have midface hypoplasia (relative undergrowth of the middle of the face), which predisposes them to obstructive sleep apnea. Third, children with achondroplasia may have differences in spine shape or chest wall shape, which can decrease their ability to take deep breaths and result in hypoventilation (buildup of CO_2 levels). If a child with achondroplasia is found to have significant sleep apnea, your doctor may obtain imaging of the head and neck (CT or MRI) to evaluate for brain stem compression that may require surgical correction. In addition, obstructive sleep apnea can be managed with adenotonsillectomy, CPAP, supplemental oxygen, or tracheostomy depending on the particular child.

Epilepsy

Children with recurrent seizures (epilepsy) are at increased risk of sleep apnea. In addition, children with more severe epilepsy tend to have higher rates of sleep apnea compared to children with mild epilepsy[5]. Sleep apnea may cause disrupted sleep, which can then lead to increased seizure frequency. Most importantly, treating sleep apnea has been shown to reduce seizure frequency[6].

22q11 deletion syndrome

Children with 22q11 are at increased risk for sleep apnea, with approximately 50% of those undergoing a sleep study having sleep apnea[7].

Surgical treatment of sleep apnea in children with 22q11 is complicated by the fact that many of these children also have velopharyngeal insufficiency, or VPI (which is when the soft palate does not completely close against the back of the throat creating hypernasal speech). Surgical correction of VPI with placement of a pharyngeal flap can potentially worsen sleep apnea. Removal of the tonsils and adenoids can decrease severity of sleep apnea. However, removal of the adenoids in that situation can potentially worsen or cause VPI. Your surgeon will likely take all of these factors into account and discuss if removing the tonsils or adenoids would be beneficial in your child's case or not.

Infants

Just like older children, infants can have sleep apnea. In fact, they can be born with obstructive sleep apnea. Most of these infants have underlying craniofacial or congenital medical conditions such as Pierre Robin sequence. The most common reasons for obstructive sleep apnea in infants is a smaller jaw (as in Pierre Robin sequence) and laryngomalacia (a floppy voice box). Options to treat sleep apnea in infants include oxygen treatment using a nasal cannula, CPAP therapy and surgery such as supraglottoplasty (see Chapters 4 and 5). Infants with Pierre Robin and obstructive sleep apnea may undergo mandibular distraction, whereby the lower jaw and associated soft tissue (such as the tongue) are gradually moved forward to relieve airway obstruction; this procedure may help avoid tracheostomy in many of these children.

In addition to obstructive sleep apnea, infants can have central sleep apnea. It is common for infants to have some degree of periodic breathing (irregular breathing), but if it is too frequent this can disrupt sleep and affect growth and development. Your doctor many order additional tests to rule out underlying reasons for central sleep apnea. Treatment options for central sleep apnea include supplemental oxygen or medications that stimulate breathing. Many infants, as they grow older and their brain matures and airway enlarges, can grow out of their sleep apnea.

Neuromuscular patients

Children with neuromuscular conditions are at increased risk for two potential sleep conditions that can occur simultaneously. First, their weaker upper respiratory muscles can increase their risk for obstructive sleep apnea or collapse of the upper airway during sleep. Because their muscles are weaker, they do not always have the loud snoring that is typically seen in this disorder. Instead, they can have frequent awakenings, choking noted in their sleep, restless sleep, frequent headaches upon awakening that resolve within 10-15 minutes of being awake, and increased daytime drowsiness. If these symptoms develop, it is important to tell your physician.

Patients with neuromuscular weakness are also at risk for alveolar hypoventilation. People with alveolar hypoventilation cannot take deep enough breaths to get in the needed oxygen to keep their oxygen saturations in the high 90s and remove the carbon dioxide from the body. Persistently low oxygen saturations can stress the heart in any individual; however, in many neuromuscular conditions the heart is already compromised with cardiomyopathy (disease of the heart muscle) can be present. High carbon dioxide levels can stop a child's breathing, so management of this is critical.

Finding underlying sleep-disordered breathing is important for many reasons in this population. Since breathing against a set continuous positive pressure (CPAP) can tire out children with an underlying neuromuscular condition, it is important that an inspiratory pressure to further support them is also started. This two-pressure system, also called bi-level ventilation, is delivered with a BPAP machine. Even young children with a neuromuscular condition who are still ambulatory and only have obstructive sleep apnea are started on bi-level non-invasive ventilator support (BPAP) for this reason. It is also critical to set a rate on the BPAP machine. This means that if the child becomes too weak to trigger the BPAP machine, the machine will give a mandatory amount of breaths each minute to make sure adequate ventilation occurs. A child's muscle strength varies significantly from when a child is well or acutely sick. He may be able to trigger the BPAP machine when well, but this may not be the case when ill; therefore, setting a rate is critical for the safety of the neuromuscular patient on BPAP support.

Of all the different types of bi-phasic non-invasive ventilator support used, BPAP AVAPS is the most common one prescribed for older children, because it can adjust the inspiratory pressure given to the child based on measured volumes of air that are exhaled, ensuring that adequate amounts of air are given over time. As a child gets ill, the inspiratory pressure may need to be higher for a period of time. But as the illness resolves, the inspiratory pressure can be decreased. The BPAP AVAPS setting will automatically adjust (making small changes on its own within the parameters your physician has set for it) ensuring that your child is well-ventilated even when ill with a minor respiratory illness. If the machine reaches its highest settings and still cannot deliver the recommended volume of air, it will sound an alarm. Sometimes hospitalization is required with severe respiratory illnesses.

References

1. Friedman NR, Ruiz AG, Gao D, Ingram DG. Accuracy of Parental Perception of Nighttime Breathing in Children with Down Syndrome. Otolaryngol Head Neck Surg. 2017 Sep 1:194599817726286.

2. Ingram DG, Ruiz AG, Gao D, Friedman NR. Success of Tonsillectomy for Obstructive Sleep Apnea in Children With Down Syndrome. J Clin Sleep Med. 2017 Aug 15;13(8):975-980.

3. Sedky K, Bennett DS, Pumariega A. Prader Willi syndrome and obstructive sleep apnea: co-occurrence in the pediatric population. J Clin Sleep Med. 2014 Apr 15;10(4):403-9.

4. DelRosso LM, Gonzalez-Toledo E, Hoque R. A three-month-old achondroplastic baby with both obstructive apneas and central apneas. J Clin Sleep Med. 2013 Mar 15;9(3):287-9.

5. Jain SV, Simakajornboon S, Shapiro SM, et al. Obstructive sleep apnea in children with epilepsy: prospective pilot trial. Acta Neurol Scand. 2012 Jan;125(1):e3-6

6. Gogou M, Haidopoulou K, Eboriadou M, Paylou E. Sleep apneas and epilepsy comorbidity in childhood: a systematic review of the literature. Sleep Breath. 2015 May;19(2):421-32.

7. Kennedy WP1, Mudd PA2, Maguire MA3, et al. 22q11.2 Deletion syndrome and obstructive sleep apnea. Int J Pediatr Otorhinolaryngol. 2014 Aug;78(8):1360-4.

9

ADDITIONAL RESOURCES FOR PARENTS

sleepapnea.org

The American Sleep Apnea Association (ASAA) is a nonprofit organization that works to improve awareness of sleep apnea and advocate for sleep apnea patients. Their website features educational materials as well as a CPAP assistance program.

babysleep.com

Babysleep.com is an excellent resource for up-to-date and accurate information on sleep in young children. The website was developed and is maintained by the Pediatric Sleep Council, an international group of pediatric sleep experts, and features general advice as well as tips for specific sleep issues. One very nice feature of this website is video interviews of pediatric sleep experts. Finally, this website features a search engine to find an AASM-accredited sleep center that specializes in treatment of young children.

sleepeducation.org

The American Academy of Sleep Medicine (AASM) is the major professional organization in sleep medicine. Their educational website at sleepeducation.org has several educational materials and articles regarding sleep apnea and other sleep disorders. You can also search for an accredited sleep center on their site.

sleep.org

The National Sleep Foundation (NSF) is a nonprofit organization that educates the public regarding sleep health.

entnet.org

The website of the American Academy of Otolaryngology-Head and Neck Surgery features wonderful educational materials regarding sleep apnea as well as other ENT conditions, and you can search for ENT physicians specializing in pediatrics based on your location.

Sleeping Through the Night: How Infants, Toddlers, and Their Parents Can Get a Good Night's Sleep.

This is a wonderful book detailing tips and techniques for dealing with common behavioral sleep problems in infants and young children.

American Academy of Dental Sleep Medicine.

The AADSM website at aadsm.org features several patient resources, including resources on searching for an AADSM dentist and educational materials regarding oral appliance therapy.

Johnson's Bedtime baby sleep app.

This free app was developed by pediatric sleep experts in conjunction with Johnson & Johnson. The app allows you to track your young child's sleep, have your sleep questions answered by experts, and also features a playlist of lullabies and ambient sounds.

The Toddler Owner's Manual: Operating Instructions, Troubleshooting Tips, and Advice on System Maintenance.

A wonderful book by Brett Kuhn and colleagues featuring instructions, tips, and tricks for toddler care, including behavioral challenges.

sleepapnea.com

This website produced by Phillips Respironics features many educational videos as well as resources regarding specific Respironics machines.

iaom.com

The website for the International Association of Orofacial Myology includes educational materials regarding myofunctional therapy as well as the ability to search for certified providers.

nichd.nih.gov/sts/

This Safe to Sleep resource from the Eunice Kennedy Shriver National Institute of Child Health and Human Development provides excellent educational resources regarding safe infant sleep habits to prevent sudden infant death syndrome (SIDS). Free resources are available in online, print, and video formats.

ndss.org

The National Down Syndrome Society has a plethora of resources for families with children who have Down syndrome, including educational resources, a helpline, local support groups, and advocacy projects.

pwsausa.org

The Prader-Willi Syndrome Association provides support to families of children with PWS. The organization provides emotional support to families, encourages research, educates regarding the condition, and advocates for patients.

lpaonline.org

Little People of America is a nonprofit organization dedicated to people with dwarfism and their families. They provide support, education, scholarships, and a newsletter.

22q.org

The International 22q11.2 Foundation supports the detection, care, and efforts at finding a cure for 22q. Their overall mission is to improve quality of life for individuals affected by 22q.

ABOUT THE EDITOR

David Ingram, MD, is a board-certified pediatrician and sleep physician at Children's Mercy Hospital. He completed his pediatric residency at the University of Wisconsin-Madison and sleep medicine fellowship at the University of Colorado and National Jewish Health. He currently serves as a founding editor of the Pediatric Sleep Case Conference as well as president-elect of the Missouri Sleep Society. He is assistant professor of pediatrics, and adjunct assistant professor in the department of psychology where he teaches a Sleep & Dreams college course at the University of Missouri-Kansas City. He lives in Parkville, Missouri with his wife and daughter.

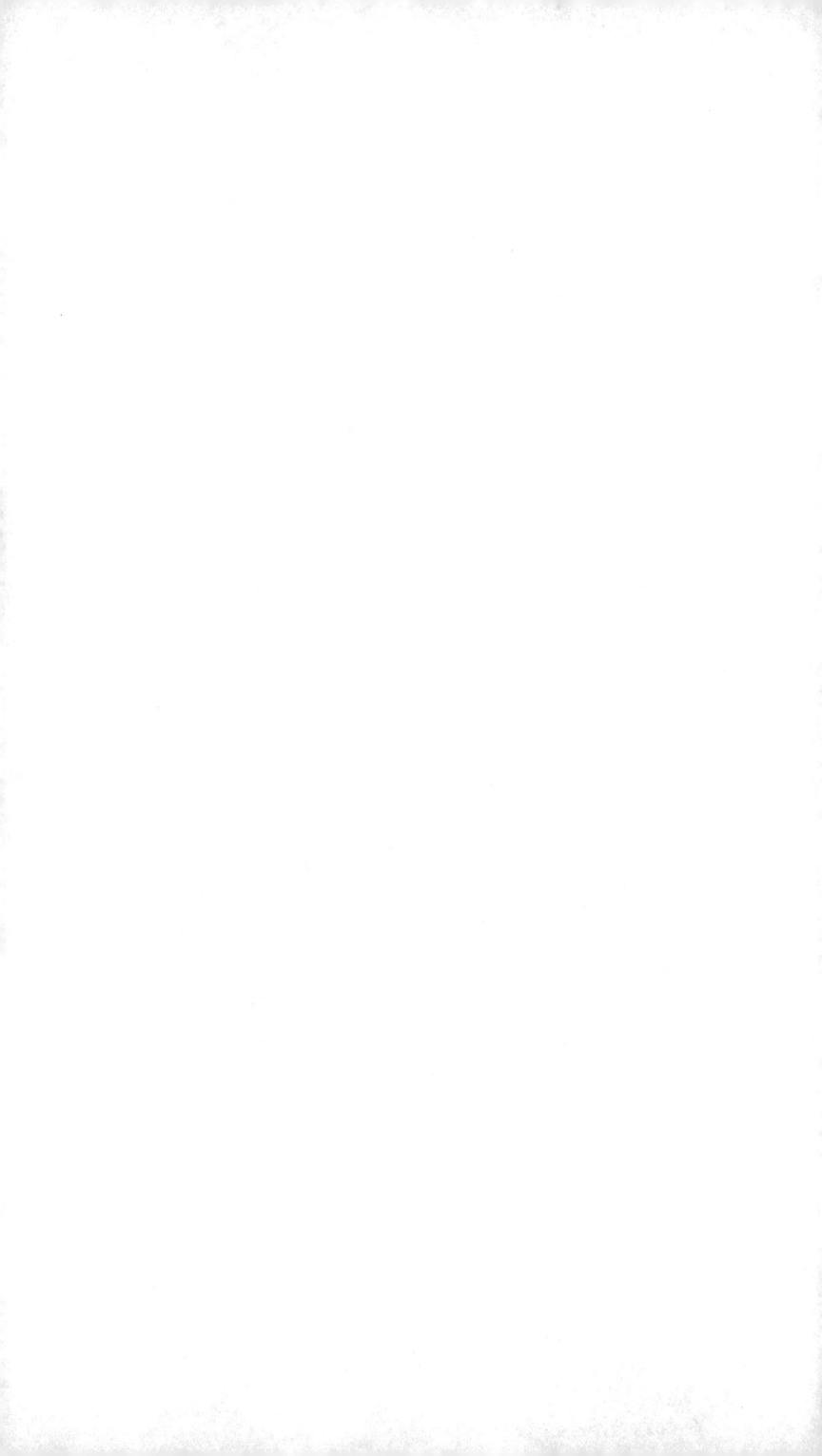